Optimal Muscle
Performance
and Recovery

"A more informed athlete is a better athlete. Thanks to Dr. Ed Burke, we are no longer in the dark about how to maximize performance. The science of recovery has been taken to a new level. This book gives athletes the advantage they need to win."

ALISON DUNLAP, *2001 world mountain bike champion, and 2002 World Cup mountain bike champion*

"Dr. Ed Burke has made a major contribution to the science of recovery. He outlines in a very understandable fashion the current body of scientific knowledge with regard to renewing muscle fibers. His four simple principles, incorporated into the R^4 System, explain the process. It's not magic—it's scientifically based and it makes sense."

FRANK SHORTER, *Olympic Marathon gold and silver medalist*

"It is no longer enough to train hard—recovery is emerging as the real key to athletic improvement. Ed Burke's new book shows you how to take maximum advantage of those grueling workouts with world-class recovery techniques."

FRED MATHENY, *fitness editor for www.roadbikerider.com*

"Ed Burke unveils the latest clinical yet practical nutritional truths about muscle recovery. The book will be an invaluable training and racing tool for all athletes and coaches who have questioned the validity of optimum dietary supplementation to enhance performance. *Optimal Muscle Performance and Recovery* is a fantastic addition to my health library."

DAVE SCOTT, *six-time winner of the Ironman Triathlon*

"A simple but dramatic approach to improved training, fitness, and recovery that anyone can follow on a daily basis. Highly recommended."

BOB ANDERSON, *author of* Stretching

"*Optimal Muscle Performance and Recovery* is a must for coaches and athletes. It contains a lot of important information on how to maximize your training and excel in your sport. The book makes you understand how important recovery is for your athletic success. I wish this kind of knowledge had been available when I was competing."

GRETE WAITZ, *nine-time winner of the New York City Marathon*

"Recovery, often neglected by both the recreational and elite athlete, is one of the keys to continual improvement in sport. In *Optimal Muscle Performance and Recovery*, Ed Burke shows the reader how and why to utilize the R^4 System of recovery for improved athletic success. What could be easier? If you want to train and compete at a higher level, read this book and put it to use."

HARVEY NEWTON, CSCS, *former Executive Director of NSCA;*
National Strength and Conditioning Coach,
USA Weightlifting Team, 1984 Olympic Games

"This is the most comprehensive book I've read on the topic of nutrition for muscle performance and recovery, written for both endurance and team sports athletes. It is filled with practical information that is backed up with scientific research. Everyone from the weekend warrior to the serious athlete will benefit from reading this book."

PAUL GOLDBERG, R.D., CSCS, *strength and conditioning coach*
for the Colorado Avalanche hockey team

"Ed Burke has done it again! This new edition is packed with practical, user-friendly information on sports nutrition. Balanced, authoritative, and scientifically sound, this is a must-read for all who want to improve."

RICK CURL, *head coach, Curl-Burke Swim Club,*
seven-time USA swimming national team champion

Optimal Muscle Performance and Recovery

USING THE REVOLUTIONARY R⁴ SYSTEM® TO REPAIR
AND REPLENISH MUSCLES FOR PEAK PERFORMANCE

Edmund R. Burke, Ph.D.

A V E R Y
a member of Penguin Putnam Inc.
New York

Most Avery books are available at special quantity discounts for bulk purchase for sales promotions, premiums, fund-raising, and educational needs. Special books or book excerpts also can be created to fit specific needs. For details, write Putnam Special Markets, 375 Hudson Street, New York, NY 10014.

a member of
Penguin Putnam Inc.
375 Hudson Street
New York, NY 10014
www.penguinputnam.com

Library of Congress Cataloging-in-Publication Data

Burke, Edmund, date.
[Optimal muscle recovery]
Optimal muscle performance and recovery : using the Revolutionary R^4 System
to repair and replenish muscles for peak performance / Edmund R. Burke.
p. cm.
Originally published as Optimal muscle recovery.
Includes bibliographical references and index.
ISBN 1-58333-146-8
1. Physical fitness. 2. Physical fitness—Nutritional aspects. 3. Muscles—
Motility—Nutritional aspects. 4. Diet. I. Title.
RA781 .B876 2003
613.7—dc21
2002038556

Printed in the United States of America
1   3   5   7   9   10   8   6   4   2

Book design by Amanda Dewey

CONTENTS

Acknowledgments   ix

Foreword to the First Edition   xi

Foreword to the Second Edition   xiii

Introduction   I

Part I: Muscle Performance Basics   9

1. How Muscles Work   I I

2. The Energy Currency of Muscles   18

3. What Causes Muscle Fatigue?   29

4. What Causes Muscle Soreness?   45

5. Recovery: Your Key to Peak Performance   53

Part II: The R⁴ System for Peak Performance   63

6. Refuel and Rehydrate Muscles During Exercise   65

7. Replenish Glycogen After Exercise   91

8. Reduce Muscle and Immune-System Stress   100

9. Rebuild Muscle Protein   114

10. Making Science Practical: The R⁴ Recovery System   122

Part III: Going the Extra Mile   133

11. Optimal Recovery for the Strength Athlete   135

12. Recovery for the Masters Athlete   149

13. Nutrition for Every Day   160

14. Vitamins and Minerals: Keys to Improved Performance   180

15. Enhancing Performance, Reducing Injuries, and Improving Recovery with Sports Supplements   197

16. Nutrition to Delay Event Fatigue   215

17. Sleep and Recovery   226

18. Nonnutritional Approaches to Recovery   238

Conclusion   253

Glossary   257

References   262

Index   283

ACKNOWLEDGMENTS

I am grateful to the many dedicated people whose hard work and support made this project possible. First, thanks to Robert Portman, Ph.D., for hosting and supporting the symposium that led to the creation of this book. It was obvious after listening to the guest speakers that there was a better nutritional regimen to help athletes improve athletic performance.

I would like to thank Drs. John Ivy and Robert Kaman, as well as Dr. Portman, for their careful critiquing and editing of the book. Thanks also to Drs. John Seifert and Peter Raven, and to all the students in their laboratories who worked on the research presented in this book.

I would also like to thank the good people at Avery of Penguin Putnam, and in particular the editor of the first edition, Peggy Hahn, and the editor of the second edition, Carol Rosenberg. Without their steady and professional editorial hands to guide and shape the final presentation of each version of the manuscript, this book would never have come to fruition.

My deepest gratitude goes out to all the athletes I have worked with over the last twenty years, who have given me the insight to look beyond "traditional" nutritional information and research to find the truth behind sports nutrition. I am also indebted to the many scientists, nutritionists, and medical professionals who are expanding the frontiers of our knowledge of nutrition, antioxidants, herbs, and carbohydrate/protein supplementation. We are very fortunate to have these dedicated men and women waging the war against complacency in nutrition research and education.

Above all, I am thankful to have a wonderful wife, Kathleen, who understands the long hours it takes to write books of this nature. She has always been there to support my efforts.

There are many others, too numerous to name, who have guided, advised, and supported me as I put this book together. I owe them all a debt of gratitude for helping me to produce a guide that will be helpful to you, my reader, and to the athletes you work with on the field or in the gym.

We all want to get the most out of our training programs. Some of us exercise for fitness, others train for competition, but all of us push our bodies to the limit—sometimes daily—in order to maximize our workouts. As dedicated athletes, we may put in several hours at a time of strenuous exercise to improve beyond basic conditioning and develop strength and endurance. But intense, exhaustive exercise is only one aspect of an effective training program.

Successful athletes and their coaches and trainers know that it's impossible to train extremely hard on consecutive days for any extended period of time. This is especially true for endurance runners. Our bodies need approximately twenty-four to thirty-six hours to recover from strenuous training. Nowadays, a "hard-easy" schedule, which incorporates easy days of less intense training, is an accepted part of every smart endurance athlete's routine. It's as simple as listening to your body. You know when you have maximized your workout or raced to your limit because your body will not allow you to continue, and you won't be able to go at the same level the next day—no matter how hard you try.

Optimal Muscle Recovery is a breakthrough contribution to the science of recovery from exercise. For years now, we have been aware of the importance of replacement drinks to restore the body's needed levels of fluids (such as water) and salts (such as sodium, potassium, and magnesium). Dr. Edmund Burke has taken the idea of restoring balance to a new level. In this book, he teaches us that returning to a state of balance also involves replenishing energy stores and rebuilding damaged muscle fibers. With his revolutionary R^4 System, Dr. Burke has interpreted the current body of scientific knowledge into four remarkably simple principles that will help you to maximize your recovery from exercise. The secret to complete recovery lies in carefully balanced nutrition and nutritional supplementation that will enable you to reduce muscle damage, restore energy, and regain your strength after exercise. When you help your body make a full recovery, you'll find that it's easier to exercise at peak capacity in your next training session.

Reaching your performance goals takes time and a great deal of patience. You can't "magically" achieve the standards that you set for yourself without hard work and perseverance. But *Optimal Muscle Recovery* presents real-world, practical guidelines that can help you get started on the road to peak performance.

—Frank Shorter
Olympic Marathon Champion

Most people involved with sports medicine have a sport that is of prime interest, and mine is soccer. While playing in college, I realized that my ticket to a starting position was going to be my overall fitness level. In the early 1970s, I participated in an exercise physiology study and was lucky to have been influenced by a man who was interested in performance. He explained to me that "performance" basically meant how well your body responds to what you ask it to do.

As a result, my old prof and I put together a summer training program designed to enhance my fitness level through performance and recovery. Specifically, our goal was to improve my ability to perform *lots* of runs separated by short recovery periods. So while most other athletes were concentrating on fitness trends at that time, like maximal oxygen consumption and distance running, I became interested in this concept of recovery—including both recovery between runs *and* recovery between exercise sessions or competitions.

Improvements in physical training have resulted in soccer being played at a much faster level than when I played in college. The running volume in soccer has gone up around 20 percent or more for the same 90-minute game on the same size field. Running distances for the men's game in the early '70s are what is expected of today's female players, with some women covering distances very close to that of men.

Achieving this increased level of fitness and performance isn't easy. Training hard for longer periods of time *and* for more days each week requires an improved understanding of what the body must do *between* sessions to be prepared for the *next* training bout. Just what does the body have to do to refuel, repair, and rebuild in order to be ready to go at it again? The vast majority of books and articles available to the practicing athlete and coach discuss only the actual training, giving short shrift to the recovery period between workouts that is as essential to training as the workout itself.

Dr. Burke's career has been focused on making sure that the athlete is prepared fully for competition, giving special consideration to how the body recovers between exercise sessions in order to achieve optimal training levels. His book, *Optimal Muscle Performance and Recovery*, outlines his approach to training as well as to the all-important recovery period. The coach who ignores the concepts of performance and recovery will be putting his or her charges at a competitive disadvantage compared to the coach who incorporates the latest findings from this exciting branch of sports medicine.

—Don Kirkendall, Ph.D.
   Member, U.S. Soccer Sports Medicine, Physical Fitness and Research
   Committee; Assistant Professor, Department of Orthopaedics,
   University of North Carolina

INTRODUCTION

I started to study exercise physiology and sports nutrition in the 1970s with the conviction that proper nutrition, in addition to a good training program, is crucial for optimal performance. In the years since then, I have had the good fortune to work with a number of the world's leading sports scientists and to collaborate with them on studies that have defined a new vision of sports nutrition.

Much of the research conducted in the last three decades has focused on gaining a greater understanding of the body's physiological responses to dehydration and of the impact of carbohydrate supplementation—prior to and during exercise—on performance. Studies on carbohydrate, in particular, have highlighted the effects of pre-exercise energy stores on endurance performance, which has resulted in a popular practice known as *carbohydrate loading.* Sports scientists and nutritionists have also investigated the roles of other basic nutrients, such as protein and fat, in fueling exercise. The culmination of this research has been the establishment of guidelines for an effective athletic diet.

Only in the last few years, however, have we begun to investigate the role of nutrition in helping muscles to recover from exercise that lasts more than sixty minutes, which is generally referred to as *long-term exercise*. Because most of your muscles' adaptations for increased strength and endurance occur in the interval between exercise sessions, your ability to perform at a high level day after day is limited by the extent of muscle recovery and repair after strenuous training. Therefore, it's no longer enough to train long and hard—you have to train smart.

"Take rest and recovery nutrition as seriously as you take your training," says Jay T. Kearney, Ph.D., former director of Sports Science at the Olympic Training Center in Colorado Springs, Colorado. "For the most part, strength and endurance capacity are developed not during the training session but instead during the rest phase, when the muscle tissue grows stronger." It has become quite clear that providing the right nutrients in the right proportions before, during, and after exercise ensures your muscles' health and increases endurance capacity and strength, all of which lead to improved performance. Not only should you replenish your body's depleted energy stores, but you also have to take steps to minimize and repair damaged muscle tissue. Sports nutrition research now provides us with guidance to achieve this goal.

THE R⁴ SYSTEM OF RECOVERY

Several years ago, I participated in a symposium in Colorado Springs, attended by top exercise physiologists. The objective of the symposium was to review the most recent studies on enhancing recovery both during and after exercise. It was during this symposium that the R⁴ System for Peak Performance was developed, with the basic goal to help athletes achieve full muscle potential through a comprehensive recovery program.

Based on the latest research on muscle performance and recovery, the R⁴ System is an important milestone in our understanding of exercise physiology. It highlights the importance of energy replacement during and after exercise to extend performance, and it focuses on minimizing and repairing exercise-induced muscle damage in order to maintain muscle strength. The R^4 System establishes four simple, practical principles that all endurance athletes can incorporate into their daily training. If you want to optimize recovery and achieve full muscle potential, you should:

- **Refuel** and rehydrate muscles during and after exercise.
- **Replenish** glycogen, a primary fuel source for energy.
- **Reduce** muscle and immune-system damage resulting from the physical stress of exercise.
- **Rebuild** muscle protein, which is important for the maintenance of muscle structure and function.

Part I of *Optimal Muscle Performance and Recovery* lays the groundwork in clear, understandable terms by reviewing basic muscle structure and function. You'll learn about the essential nutrients that your body uses for energy, and the three possible ways in which your muscles "burn" these nutrients for fuel. This is followed by a comprehensive look at the causes of muscle fatigue and exercise-induced muscle damage. Finally, Part I establishes the foundation for the R^4 System by explaining the processes involved in recovery from exercise.

A NEW MODEL FOR SPORTS PERFORMANCE

In addition to recovery, how one hydrates and fuels one's muscles during exercise is also undergoing a renaissance. Only a few years ago, the idea of combining carbohydrate with protein during exercise in a sports drink in an optimal ratio was born. This has been gaining in popularity among endurance athletes ever since. This trend is a result of the growing body of data documenting the synergism of protein/carbohydrate mixtures. Protein-containing sports drinks are indeed a major breakthrough in the way sports drinks can enhance performance.

Comparing the labels of sports drinks gives the impression that the only feature that differentiates drinks is taste. All you have to do is throw some various types of carbohydrate into water, toss in a few electrolytes, add flavor, and you have a new-generation sports drink, right? The answer is both yes and no. Yes, a number of products are simply carbohydrate, salt-and-pepper amounts of electrolytes, and flavor. And no, as you will soon see from new and convincing research that a well-designed sports drink should contain nutrients other than the aforementioned.

Most during-exercise sports products available today focus primarily on rehydration and carbohydrate supplementation. These products are based on thirty-year-old science and ignore the importance of stimulating the hormone insulin via protein intake with carbohydrate, thereby improving glucose uptake by (or glucose delivery to) the muscle and reducing muscle and oxidative stress. Manufacturers of products that contain protein have taken the approach that more is better. Research has shown that the opposite is true. Although protein plays a critical role in the rebuilding of damaged muscle and the glycogen replenishment process, too much protein will slow hydration and gastric emptying (the rate at which your stomach contents are emptied into the intestines). The ratio of carbohydrate to protein that is most desirable is 4 to 1. At this ratio, the combination of nutrients delivers the benefits of protein without negatively impacting the critical rehydration process. This book examines some of the research that has been conducted in the last few years that establishes the 4-to-1 ratio as a model that explains the interaction of key physiological and nutritional factors that enable muscles to operate at peak levels.

PUTTING SCIENCE INTO PRACTICE

Part II is the heart of the book because it details each of the four components of the R^4 System. It discusses the research behind the development of an energy/hydration sports-drink system that combines both carbohydrate and protein, which represents an important advance in sports-drink research. The combining of carbohydrate and protein in a 4-to-1 ratio enables endurance athletes to uptake more glucose by the active muscles during exercise, resulting in improved energy production, sparing of muscle glycogen, and extended endurance in the later stages of competition. The bottom line is that you can train and compete longer and harder. With the introduction of a 4-to-1 carbohydrate/protein ratio, sports drinks have entered a new era in optimizing athletic performance.

Since the publication of the first edition of this book, several sports nutritional beverages have been introduced to the sports nutrition market based on the 4-to-1 ratio. Other products using ratios ranging from 3-to-1 to 5-to-1 have also been produced. My recommendation of the 4-to-1 ratio is based on a review of data on performance and recovery published in the scientific literature and also on research that I have participated in over the last five years.

Whether you use a 4-to-1 ratio of carbohydrate/protein or a modification of this ratio, you will experience further gains in performance and muscle recovery. The key is the proper balance of water, carbohydrate, protein, essential amino acids, and antioxidants that exist in this new generation of sports and recovery drinks.

In this book, you'll discover how to maximize recovery by making some surprisingly simple changes in your exercise-nutrition program. And each chapter in Part II provides you with guidelines that will enable you to tailor these revolutionary nutritional principles to suit your body's needs. This part of the book also explains how exercise physiologists have made science practical by developing a new sports nutrition product based upon the latest research on recovery.

GOING THE EXTRA MILE

Part III of *Optimal Muscle Performance and Recovery* takes you beyond the R^4 System by outlining other measures that will help you enhance performance and maintain overall health. This part provides an overview of general nutrition for maximal performance in your everyday activities, even when you're not exercising. Following this is a discussion of cutting-edge nutritional supplements that athletes who are "in the know" are using to optimize recovery, from the well-known creatine and caffeine to the lesser known phosphatidylserine. This final part also shows you how to stockpile your energy stores through carbohydrate loading prior to intense exercise or competition—without suffering from common side effects such as heaviness in the limbs. Last but not least, you'll find important information on nonnutritional approaches to recovery, from sleep, stretching, and pre- and post-competition massage to sessions in the sauna or hot tub.

SPORTS NUTRITION: HOW MUCH RESEARCH IS ENOUGH?

As with any book about sports nutrition and supplementation, a healthy dose of criticism always follows. Yes, I know that the data are still incomplete in the areas of sports drinks, supplements, and recovery beverages. Yes, I know that they are often inconclusive. And yes, I know that more data are needed.

Does that mean I should hide in my ivory tower and refrain from giving practical advice to athletes? I think not. Yet, from my experience, that seems to be the case with many scientists. As a scientist, I am often caught between athletes seeking practical advice and scientists who are very disinclined to give an opinion regarding supplementation other than "eat a balanced diet and drink plenty of water." Or, there never seems to be enough articles published in the scientific literature to totally convince these scientists that a nutrient works physiologically. In fact, several of my colleagues subscribe to the notion that taking recovery drinks and supplements is largely ineffectual, costly, and a waste of time. Yet, go to any supermarket and you will find orange juice fortified with vitamin C and calcium. You will also find refined bread fortified with B vitamins, milk fortified with vitamin D, and so on. There is even sports water fortified with antioxidants.

So why does the use of some dietary supplements and energy foods by athletes provoke such a negative response? As a scientist, I do not believe it is wrong to provide opinions based on incomplete data. If scientists are the "experts" from whom the public seeks advice, then should I not provide such information? Or should I leave that to the scientist who believes only in the literature and who has never worked with athletes or competed himself? Remember, for years, many scientists said that we only needed water during exercise, that protein intake above the RDA was unhealthy, that antioxidants serve no protective purpose, and on and on. From whom would you seek advice? How long do we wait for the definitive answer? For some, no amount of papers published in the scientific literature will ever convince them that a nutritional supplement, type of drink, and so on could ever improve athletic performance.

I realize that this book might contain controversial statements, but I also realize that an attempt to please everyone is a formula for failure. However, as a scientist, I realize how insular our field can be. Indeed, it is far better to try to give well-intentioned advice rather than to hide behind the clichéd "more research is needed" answer.

The goal of this book is to help you better understand how exercise affects your muscles, and how taking measures to ensure proper nutrient intake both during exercise and in recovery can improve performance and counteract some of the consequences of strenuous training or competition. You will learn how to extend performance, maintain muscle strength, and develop your muscles day by day. By adopting the R^4 System for Peak Performance, you'll feel healthier and perform at a higher level than you ever thought possible.

Optimal Muscle Performance and Recovery is designed to give you up-to-date information about sports nutrition and training in clear, easy-to-understand language. It can be read cover to cover or dipped into as necessary when information is needed on a specific topic. Based upon scientific research and documentation with more than two hundred references, it will show you how good nutrition and supplementation can help improve your performance and boost your recovery ability. Use this book as your guide to your physical best, in your health and in your sport.

Part I

Muscle Performance Basics

Whether you're a professional athlete or a "weekend warrior," you probably know what it's like to run out of steam during strenuous exercise. And maybe, the day after intense training, your sore, stiff muscles remind you that you had better take it easy next time. Most athletes accept these consequences of exercise as inevitable. Many, in fact, take these signs to mean that they are not training hard enough, and they concentrate on increasing the difficulty or duration of their workouts. The problem with this approach is that it does not address the underlying causes of muscle fatigue and soreness. Learning how to minimize these discomforts is as simple as understanding how your muscles work and how exercise affects their structure and function.

Part I reviews the mechanics and chemistry behind muscle contraction, from the physical structure of human skeletal muscle to the way your body uses carbohydrate, fat, and protein to synthesize energy for all of its activities. This part then builds upon this information to explain how exercise affects your muscles on the physical and biochemical levels, causing fatigue and muscle damage. And, most important, this part explains the three critical phases of recovery, during which time your body returns to a state of balance, replenishes depleted energy stores, and repairs damaged muscle tissue.

How Muscles Work

Many people are of the opinion that well-developed muscles are the most visible testament to physical fitness. Firm, toned muscles are aesthetically pleasing, and millions of us dedicate hours each day to exercise in an effort to appear "muscular." However, we have to look beyond size—the most obvious aspect of muscles—to understand muscular fitness. The most important aspect of our skeletal muscle system is function.

Muscles are highly specialized tissues that can contract to produce body movement. They enable us to carry out the innumerable functions that are essential to daily life. However, most people don't know about the underlying physiology of the human skeletal muscle system. This is because our actions are generated so quickly that we're not aware of the complicated processes behind them.

To understand how muscle recovery is key to peak muscle performance during exercise, you should have some background knowledge about how your muscles work. This chapter reviews basic muscle structure and function.

THE THREE TYPES OF MUSCLE CELLS

Muscle tissue makes up a large part of the human body—40 to 45 percent of a man's body by weight and 30 to 35 percent of a woman's body by weight. Of course, percentage of muscle weight is considerably higher in those athletes who train regularly and intensely, such as champion bodybuilders. In total, your body contains some 650 muscles. About 620 of these muscles are called skeletal muscles because they are fastened to the bones of your skeleton by strong connective tissues known as tendons. The main function of the skeletal muscle system is the voluntary movement of the body. These muscles are classified as voluntary muscles because you can contract them at will.

The remaining muscles are composed of cardiac muscle and smooth muscle. Cardiac muscle, or heart muscle, is responsible for pumping blood through the body. Smooth muscle is found in the walls of organs such as the stomach, intestines, and urinary bladder, and in blood vessels. Among its many other functions, smooth muscle helps substances move through the intestinal tract, and also changes the diameter of blood vessels. Because you cannot control the contractions of your smooth muscles at will, they are known as *involuntary muscles.*

THE STRUCTURE AND FUNCTION OF SKELETAL MUSCLE

Skeletal muscle tissue is composed of bundles of long fibers. Each fiber is actually a muscle cell, which is surrounded by a thin membrane. Muscle cells are responsible for producing the enormous amounts of energy that your muscles require for contraction.

Figure 1.1 on page 13 provides a closer look at the individual muscle

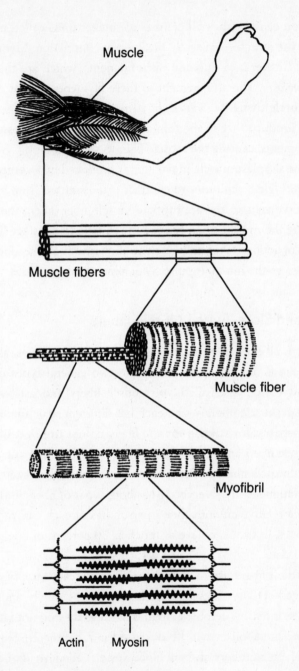

Figure 1.1. The structure of skeletal muscles

fiber. As you can see, the cell consists of smaller units called myofibrils, which are the structures directly involved in contraction. Myofibrils can be divided further into thin and thick filaments, which are the proteins *actin* and *myosin*. The arrangement of these filaments is what gives your skeletal muscle tissue its *striated*, or striped, appearance. Muscular contraction is produced when the thin actin filaments slide across the thick myosin filaments, causing the muscle fiber to shorten.

Even the simplest muscle movement is produced by a complex series of operations. First, the order to contract is transmitted from your brain by your nerve cells to the appropriate muscle fiber. Then, the stimulus passes along the muscle fiber, causing the muscle to contract. This intricate series of actions takes only one one-thousandth of a second, making the response to the initial impulse seem almost instantaneous.

Fast- and Slow-Twitch Muscle Fibers

Although all skeletal muscles share the same properties, all skeletal muscle tissue is not the same. There are two general types of muscle fibers—slow-twitch (also called type I muscle fibers) and fast-twitch (also called type II muscle fibers)—and each has different structural and functional properties. Slow-twitch muscle fibers do not tire as easily as fast-twitch muscle fibers and are therefore used for high-endurance activities. Fast-twitch muscle fibers contract more quickly than slow-twitch muscle fibers, but fatigue easily. Everybody has both types of fibers in their muscles, but the relative amount that a person has of each can vary widely. Some athletes, in fact, can have as much as 80 percent of one particular fiber type.

Slow-twitch fibers use oxygen to produce a steady supply of energy for prolonged activity. These fibers function more slowly and are well suited to less intensive aerobic activities because they do not fatigue easily. (Aerobic metabolism will be discussed in Chapter 2.) Slow-twitch fibers have large numbers of small blood vessels called *capillaries* to bring in oxygen and nutrients and to carry off waste products such as carbon dioxide. Therefore, they are advantageous for long-term training or competition. Athletes who excel at endurance sports have a higher proportion of slow-twitch fibers.

Fast-twitch fibers contract rapidly and function well anaerobically, without a steady supply of oxygen. (Anaerobic metabolism will be discussed in Chapter 2.) These are responsible for strength and speed in high-intensity, low-endurance activities that demand quick bursts of energy, such as sprinting, jumping, and shot-putting. They are also used for situations where stop-and-go movements are required, such as in basketball and volleyball. However, fast-twitch fibers fatigue quickly due to the buildup of lactic acid, a byproduct of anaerobic metabolism. Not surprisingly, athletes who excel in short-duration sports requiring a high-energy output seem to have a relatively large proportion of fast- to slow-twitch fibers.

The proportion of fast- to slow-twitch muscle fibers in your muscles is determined by genetics and is therefore fixed at birth. This means that the fiber ratio cannot be altered significantly by training. Elite athletes generally possess a greater quantity of one type of fiber. For instance, a marathon runner would possess more slow-twitch fibers than a 100-meter sprinter, while the sprinter would have a greater percentage of fast-twitch fibers. All muscle fibers, however, can respond to athletic training by improving their ability to perform.

HOW OPPOSING FORCES WORK TOGETHER

Muscles can forcefully contract, but they cannot forcefully expand. This means that when a muscle pulls a bone in one direction, it is unable to pull the bone back to its original position. For this reason, skeletal muscles function in *antagonistic*, or opposing pairs.

Figure 1.2 on page 16 illustrates how two muscles work against each other to produce movements of the human arm. As shown, the contrac-

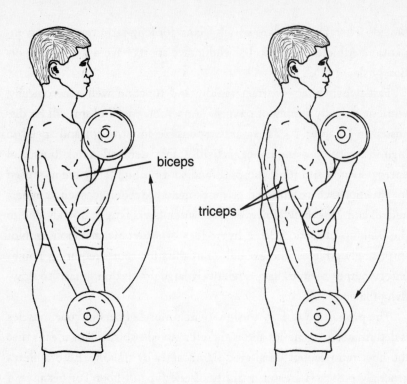

Figure 1.2. The figure on the left shows the concentric contraction of the biceps muscle, in which the biceps is the agonist, while the triceps muscle is the antagonist. The figure on the right shows the eccentric contraction of the biceps muscle, in which the triceps muscle is the agonist, and the biceps is the antagonist.

tion of your biceps muscle, which is considered to be the agonist, allows you to raise your forearm in order to lift a weight. The shortening of the biceps muscle is known as concentric contraction. At the same time, the triceps muscle, known as the antagonist, extends.

In order to lower your arm, your triceps muscle (now the agonist) must contract. This contraction allows for the relaxation and extension of the biceps muscle (now the antagonist) to return your arm to its original position. In this case, the lengthening of the biceps muscle is called *eccentric contraction*.

CONCLUSION

The architecture of your skeletal muscle system is extremely intricate. As you continue to read this book, try to notice some of the simple actions that your skeletal muscles perform—actions that you would normally take for granted, such as opening this book and turning its pages. Every movement of your body occurs through a series of precise operations that begins with the command to contract from your brain and results in the contraction of a muscle or group of muscles.

Now we can move on to examine what enables muscles to contract. The next chapter focuses on how your body produces the energy it needs for movement.

The Energy Currency of Muscles

Muscle cells require extraordinary amounts of energy to contract—especially during exercise. To produce the energy your body needs, nature has designed an extremely sophisticated metabolic system. Energy is released when your muscle cells break down carbohydrate, fat, and protein. Your body uses these nutrients in specific proportions during exercise, depending on the length and intensity of your activity.

In this chapter, we will discuss the basic nutrients that provide you with necessary energy for training or competition. We will focus on the three energy pathways by which your body "burns" these fuels to release energy for muscle contraction.

MACRONUTRIENTS

Macronutrients are nutrients that your body requires daily in large amounts in order to function properly. These nutrients, including carbohydrate, fat, and protein, supply your body with energy and serve as the building blocks for growth and repair.

The fourth and most important macronutrient, water, contains no calories (units used to measure food energy) and does not provide energy in and of itself. However, it is a vital component in every function of the body, including all digestive, absorptive, circulatory, and excretory functions. The role of this essential macronutrient will be discussed in greater detail in Chapter 3.

Carbohydrate

Carbohydrate is your body's most readily available source of nutrient energy. Through digestion and metabolism, carbohydrate (bread, vegetables, sugar, pasta, and so on) is converted into glucose to be used as an immediate source of fuel by the muscles. Glucose that is not used directly to provide energy is transported by the blood to your liver and muscle tissues, where it is converted into glycogen for storage. The hormone insulin, which is released from the pancreas, facilitates the transport of glucose from the blood to the sites of glycogen storage. However, the capacity of your liver and muscle tissues to store glycogen is limited. If you consume more carbohydrate than your body can use at that time, some carbohydrate will be stored as fat in your *adipose* (fat) tissues.

During exercise, the stored glycogen in your muscle cells is broken down into glucose to manufacture *adenosine triphosphate* (ATP), which is the ultimate source of energy for all living cells. Through proper training, athletes can "teach" their muscles to store greater amounts of glycogen and to conserve that glycogen so that they will have increased energy reserves during exercise or competition. This philosophy of training is the basis for the practice of carbohydrate loading, which will be discussed in Chapter 16.

The intensity and duration of your activity determines how much glycogen your body uses during training or competition. For example, intense activities (anaerobic) that demand a high output of energy in a short time frame, such as sprinting, quickly deplete your body's glycogen stores. Jogging, a less intense form of steady exercise, is more conservative.

Glycogen is still used, but your reserves do not run out as quickly. Keep in mind, however, that the supply will eventually be exhausted.

A nutritional concern for most individuals who exercise daily is consuming enough carbohydrate. No matter how well conditioned these athletes are, glycogen (which is stored on a limited basis) is used as a major fuel source during moderate- to high-intensity exercise. If daily carbohydrate intake is not enough to replace the muscle glycogen used during training, muscle glycogen levels drop and the athlete does not have enough fuel to train properly. Even the best-conditioned athletes can experience reduced performance and fatigue if muscle glycogen levels are below normal during periods of hard training. The same holds true for competition, as we will see in Chapter 13.

The "staleness" and general feeling of "overtraining" that you may experience during hard training may be partially due to a reduction in muscle glycogen and may be brought about by not eating enough foods high in carbohydrate. This "chronic fatigue" often keeps you from maintaining a proper training schedule and ultimately will keep you from competing at your maximal capacity.

The carbohydrate stores of an active 150-pound man total about 2,000 calories. Of these, about 1,600 calories are stored in the muscles as glycogen, where they can be used directly; 320 calories are stored in the liver as glycogen, where they can be released into the bloodstream; and about 80 calories are stored in the blood as glucose and can travel to where they are needed (including the brain, which can only burn glucose). While these numbers of calories may seem large, they will last only about two hours during high-intensity exercise.

Fat

Fat is your body's most concentrated source of food energy. Unlike the glycogen stored in your liver and muscle tissues, fat stores can fuel hours of exercise without running out. However, because the majority of fat is stored in the adipose tissue of your body, it is not as readily available for energy production as is carbohydrate. In order to be utilized for energy, fat molecules must first be broken down into fatty acids. Then, in this form, they are transported to your working muscles by the blood.

The duration of exercise directly influences how your body uses fat for energy. Fat can be broken down for energy only during low- to moderate-intensity, longer-duration aerobic exercise. Therefore, if you wish to burn fat, you will be more successful in achieving your goals by adopting a consistent, low-intensity training program.

Even if you are lean, your fat stores are large; it is not uncommon for even thin endurance athletes to have more than 40,000 calories of stored fat in their bodies.

Protein

Protein is essential for growth and development. It is a component of hormones, antibodies, enzymes, muscle, and other body tissues. Protein is also essential in the repair of cells, including muscle cells. The proteins that make up the human body are not obtained directly from the diet. Rather, dietary protein is broken down into its constituent amino acids, which the body then uses to build the specific proteins it needs. Thus, amino acids rather than protein are the essential nutrients.

Of the twenty amino acids that your body uses to make protein, eleven are designated nonessential because they can be produced by your body from other amino acids and do not need to be obtained from your diet. The other nine are essential amino acids, which your body cannot synthesize. These must be broken down from the protein that you consume in your diet. All of the essential amino acids must be present in order for your body to build or repair muscle.

The way your body uses protein during and after exercise is much more complex than the way it uses carbohydrate or fat for energy. In the hours following exercise, your body begins to build structural proteins from amino acids for muscle repair and growth, remodeling the tissues that you need for performance. This is just one reason why paying careful attention to nutrition for complete recovery should be an important part of your training program.

Again, exercise intensity and duration are important factors in deter-mining which of the nutrient fuels will be burned to energize your body. Low- to moderate-intensity exercise of long duration demands large quantities of fuel—often more than your carbohydrate and fat reserves can provide effectively. Therefore, your body begins to utilize structural and functional proteins during long-term aerobic exercise. Short-duration, high-intensity exercise, on the other hand, uses primarily glucose, so that your protein reserves are spared.

During long-term endurance exercise, your body will begin to rely on protein as one of its fuel sources. Up to 15 percent of your energy may come from protein. This is not a good state of affairs. Research will be presented in subsequent chapters showing that protein-containing sports drinks taken during exercise can help transport more glucose from the blood into the muscles and can also supply protein to offset muscle breakdown.

YOUR FITNESS LEVEL

The last factor that determines what fuel the body will burn is fitness level. When you are in good shape, the body becomes more efficient at producing energy aerobically at the same absolute intensity of effort. For example, after a few months of training, you will be able to work at a lower percentage of your maximum aerobic capacity while running, cy-cling, or swimming at the same pace or speed. This is good news to your muscle fuel stores. Now, you will be able to use more fat and less glyco-gen at the same absolute level of exercise.

When just starting an exercise program, untrained individuals begin to accumulate lactic acid in their muscles at around 60 to 70 percent of their maximal aerobic capacity. Highly trained athletes do not begin to accumulate lactic acid until about 80 to 85 percent of their maximal ca-pacity. Most often, this intensity is referred to as "anaerobic" or "lactate" threshold, and sport scientists most commonly report this value as a per-centage of one's maximal aerobic capacity.

The fitter you are, the better your muscles will use fat as the main fuel source for aerobic energy production. When you burn more fat, less stored muscle glycogen is used during exercise. In the sports nutrition world, this is known as "glycogen sparing" and plays an important role in your ability to exercise for extended periods of time.

Lastly, training allows your muscles to store more glycogen. Trained athletes are able to store about 50 percent more glycogen than untrained individuals. The good news is that increasing your fitness level allows you to store more glycogen and use more fat during exercise to spare glycogen for higher intensity efforts.

THE CHEMISTRY OF ENERGY PRODUCTION

Your body can break down carbohydrate, fat, and even protein to produce energy in three possible ways. The ATP-CP pathway and the glycolysis pathway are both forms of anaerobic metabolism, meaning that they do not require oxygen to generate ATP. Neither of these systems can use fat or protein directly as a fuel source, and therefore they rely only on carbohydrate to produce energy. Anaerobic metabolism provides energy for high-intensity exercise, such as sprinting down a basketball court or running 400 meters on a track. This energy is limited, however, lasting approximately ten seconds for the ATP-CP pathway to several minutes for glycolysis. In addition, glycolysis generates lactic acid as a byproduct. As lactic acid builds up, it slows down the ability of individual cells to produce energy, leading to muscle fatigue.

Aerobic metabolism is called into play for activities that demand a continuous supply of energy over a longer period of time, such as cross-country skiing, road cycling, swimming, and distance running. The aerobic pathway is advantageous for these types of activities because it produces a great deal more energy than anaerobic metabolism without generating lactic acid as a byproduct.

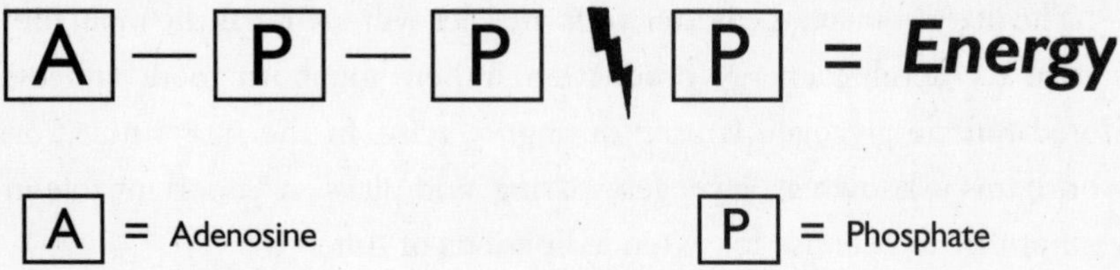

$$\boxed{A} - \boxed{P} - \boxed{P} \quad \boxed{P} = \textbf{\textit{Energy}}$$

$\boxed{A}$ = Adenosine $\boxed{P}$ = Phosphate

Figure 2.1. The release of energy from ATP

The ATP-CP Pathway

Your body uses the ATP-CP pathway to provide energy in situations requiring immediate, high-intensity actions. Because there is only enough ATP stored in your body to last for five to ten seconds of intense exercise, ATP is continually synthesized to provide energy for your muscles to function.

ATP is composed of three phosphate groups attached to an adenosine molecule by a chemical bond. The bond that connects the second and third phosphate groups is not very strong, so it is easily broken. When this occurs, a great deal of energy is released—energy that your body can then use for movement. (See Figure 2.1 above.)

When the third phosphate group is removed from ATP, the remaining molecule is *adenosine diphosphate* (ADP). This molecule can be regenerated into ATP with the help of *creatine phosphate* (CP), which acts as a phosphate storage site within your muscles. CP donates a phosphate group to ADP, creating a new molecule of ATP.

The ATP-CP cycle can continue indefinitely—as long as there's an adequate supply of creatine phosphate. When your CP reserves run low, however, your body begins to produce energy through the glycolysis pathway.

The Glycolysis Pathway

Like the ATP-CP pathway, glycolysis can occur without the presence of oxygen. In this energy pathway, stored glycogen—which is basically a long string of glucose molecules—is broken down into its glucose components. Through glycolysis, each molecule of glucose is split, and energy is released.

Glycolysis releases more energy than the ATP-CP pathway, so it is put into action when you engage in exercise that lasts from ten seconds to several minutes. But there is a disadvantage, because when there is an inadequate supply of oxygen, the glycolysis pathway produces lactic acid as a byproduct. For a time, lactic acid is quickly carried away from the muscles and returned to the liver, heart, and inactive muscles, where it is converted back into glucose. But blood and muscle concentrations begin to rise when lactic acid production proceeds at a faster pace than the speed with which it can be removed. When this occurs, you experience a burning sensation in your muscles. With a reduction in exercise intensity or a break from activity, however, the pain of lactic acid buildup generally dissipates within twenty to thirty minutes.

The Aerobic Pathway

During short-duration, high-intensity exercise, your muscles rely primarily on the ATP-CP and glycolysis pathways to produce energy. After two to three minutes, the aerobic pathway becomes the principal energy pathway, as your body begins to use oxygen to burn nutrients for energy. An important difference between the anaerobic and aerobic pathways concerns the types of nutrients that can be used to produce energy. As you can see in Figure 2.2 on page 26, the aerobic pathway uses fatty acids and amino acids in addition to glucose for energy.

Nature has established a metabolic priority system that determines when each nutrient will be mobilized as a fuel source. This system is based on the availability and efficiency with which your muscle cells can use the three nutrients. Glucose is the only fuel that can be used to produce energy in the anaerobic pathways, so it is used when there is insufficient oxygen for aerobic metabolism. Glycogen, the storage form of glucose, is found mostly in muscle and liver cells, so it can be mobilized rapidly and used as an immediate source of fuel.

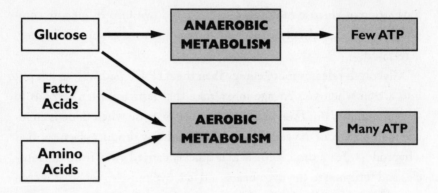

Figure 2.2. Energy production in the anaerobic and aerobic pathways

When your body shifts over to the aerobic pathway for energy production, fat is used in addition to glucose for energy. Because fat is stored mostly in the adipose tissues of the body, it is not as easily accessible as carbohydrate. It is first broken down into fatty acids before being transported to the working muscles by the blood. Your body tends to spare protein as an energy source because of its numerous other functions in the body. As explained earlier in the chapter, protein is used primarily to build and repair tissues. Therefore, protein is used only when other fuel sources begin to run low.

HOW ENDURANCE TRAINING ALTERS ENERGY PRODUCTION

Endurance training brings about a number of adaptive changes in your body. First, it increases the number of capillaries surrounding each muscle cell—sometimes by up to 40 percent. More of these small blood vessels provide for a greater exchange of oxygen and vital nutrients between the blood and the working muscle cells. Training also increases the number of red blood cells that deliver oxygen to the muscle cells. Combined, these changes help to make aerobic energy production more efficient.

Once oxygen is delivered to the cell membrane, it is transported within the cell by *myoglobin*, an iron-containing protein in muscle. Myoglobin content in skeletal muscle increases significantly following endurance training. This increase in myoglobin, however, occurs only within the muscles involved in the training and does not take place in less active muscles. Myoglobin's main function is to deliver oxygen from the cell membrane to the sites of energy production called *mitochondria*.

Aerobic energy production is the exclusive responsibility of the mitochondria. These tiny, saclike structures within your cells combine carbohydrate, fat, and protein with oxygen to produce chemical energy in the form of ATP. Within the mitochondria, the breakdown of fuels and the ultimate production of ATP depend upon the action of protein molecules called enzymes. These proteins initiate or speed chemical reactions in the body. Regular endurance training increases the number of enzymes in the mitochondria, allowing for a faster conversion of nutrient fuels into ATP. This increases the amount of energy produced in your muscle cells—and more energy means that you are able to exercise longer and at a higher intensity than are lesser trained athletes.

Muscle biopsy studies have shown that there are two major changes associated with mitochondrial energy production following endurance training: an increase in both the number and the size of the mitochondria. Research has shown a progressive weekly increase in the number of muscle mitochondria over a six-month period of endurance training. These steady but gradual changes in mitochondria suggest that the structural improvements associated with endurance training may take months and perhaps years to fully develop.

All individuals who train with the same duration and intensity will show similar adaptations in muscle, regardless of their innate talents. Despite the variety of changes that occur in the muscles during training, the adaptations that elite athletes experience are very similar to those seen in athletes who train for local races without ever winning a gold medal. Champions are born with "good genes," but they still have to put in the long hours of training to achieve their full potential.

CONCLUSION

In order for your muscles to carry out the essential processes involved in contraction, they must be able to generate energy from the macronutrients that you consume in the form of food and nutritional supplements. Through digestion and metabolism, carbohydrate, fat, and protein are broken down into smaller molecules of glucose, fatty acids, and amino acids, respectively. Your body "burns" these fuels—with or without oxygen—to generate energy in the form of ATP for muscle contraction.

Endurance training enhances the environment for energy production by increasing the amount of ATP produced in your muscles. But training alone does not guarantee optimal performance. Chapter 3 examines the six factors that can cause muscle fatigue and will guide you in learning to recognize and avoid them.

3

What Causes Muscle Fatigue?

As a sports scientist, I've had the opportunity to participate in a great deal of research concerning the causes of "hitting the wall," or "getting the bonk." Any athlete who has experienced this extreme muscle fatigue knows that it can make crossing the finish line a difficult—if not impossible—goal to achieve. Numerous studies have pointed to dehydration and carbohydrate depletion as the causes of exercise-induced fatigue. To some extent, this is true.

Today, endurance athletes know that they can prolong activity by practicing carbohydrate loading (discussed in Chapter 16) prior to extended training sessions or long competitive events. They are also aware of the importance of drinking fluids before and during exercise to prevent dehydration and heat-related illness. However, many athletes—professional or otherwise—do not know the full extent of what causes muscle fatigue. This chapter explores several other factors that contribute to fatigue, including depletion of muscle fuels, low blood glucose, increased lactic acid levels, and central fatigue.

DEHYDRATION

As stated in Chapter 2, water is an essential macronutrient in every function of the body. During exercise, it's important to make sure that you drink water because of its vital role in cardiovascular function and temperature regulation.

Heat exchange between you and the environment occurs in four ways. While cycling or running into the wind, convective cooling occurs as your body moves through the air. During swimming, excessive body heat can be lost by conduction—heat is conducted from your body to the cooler water. Heat can also be lost by radiation, provided that your body temperature is greater than the temperature of your surrounding environment.

When you exercise, your body loses water through sweating and evaporation. Sweat is your body's coolant. During an intense workout, your muscles generate heat, which is carried by your blood through capillaries near the surface of your skin. Your sweat glands release perspiration, which evaporates, cooling the skin and the blood just underneath. Cooled blood then flows back to cool your body's core.

Sweating is therefore an essential mechanism for regulating body temperature. However, when your body loses water, it limits the capacity of your blood to carry vital nutrients, such as glucose, fatty acids, and oxygen, to working muscles. The capacity of the blood to remove the byproducts of metabolism, including carbon dioxide and lactic acid, is compromised as well. The result is an increased demand on the circulatory system, which is approximately 70 percent water.

I have seen some cyclists set out for a fifty- to seventy-five-mile ride with only two small water bottles. On a hot day, the weight lost through sweat may be as much as 6 pounds. Even if a rider drinks both bicycle-style bottles, equaling about 40 ounces of water, he or she will replace only 2.5 pounds of lost fluid. In such cases, dehydration is inevitable. At the very least, this limits the cyclist's athletic performance. More seriously, it puts the athlete in jeopardy of experiencing heat-related illness and even circulatory collapse. On very long rides, runs, or hikes, use a back-mounted hydration system, such as the CamelBak Hydration System, to take along extra fluids.

Sweating is a vital thermoregulatory response that comes at the expense of maintaining your body fluids. Unless you try to keep fluid intake in pace with your sweat loss, sweating will result in dehydration. Even a slight dehydration—as little as 2 percent of your body weight—can impair athletic performance. For example, if you weigh 150 pounds, a weight loss of 3 pounds of fluid via sweating will have an effect upon performance. Athletes must drink fluids to combat the sweat loss that naturally accompanies vigorous exercise. Although it may be impossible to offset all of the water lost through sweating, even partial replacement can minimize the risk of overheating.

Pure water is acceptable for replacing fluids during exercise that lasts about thirty to sixty minutes, but drinking water is not the best way to rehydrate during exercise that lasts more than an hour nor after exercise. To restore the body fluids that you sweat out during exercise, you should consume a beverage that contains agents such as glucose and sodium, two ingredients found in most sports or energy drinks. Glucose and sodium help maintain blood volume and aid the absorption of water into your body. These two ingredients also increase thirst, which will prompt you to continue drinking—and the more you drink, the more completely you'll restore lost body fluids.

OVERHEATING

Your temperature, normally about 98.6°F, may increase to 104°F or more during intense exercise. As explained earlier in the chapter, the circulatory system transports the heat generated by muscles to the skin to be dissipated. While a certain percentage of blood is used to regulate body temperature, large quantities of blood are still required to meet the energy and metabolic needs of working muscles. These demands may overtax the circulatory system, resulting in an inadequate removal of body heat and a corresponding rise in your body temperature.

You can run the risk of overheating even in mild weather. The threat becomes more severe when weather conditions are hot and humid. Sweat doesn't evaporate well in this sort of climate because the surrounding air is already saturated with water. Without the cooling effects of sweat evaporation, your body is unable to maintain a constant body temperature that's within normal limits. If you continue to exercise in this state, you will increase your chances of suffering from heat exhaustion.

The hazards of exercising in hot, humid conditions were made abundantly clear at the 1996 Olympic Games in Atlanta, Georgia. A cycling road race was held in unfavorable conditions on a day when temperatures exceeded 85°F with high humidity and no cloud cover. Several athletes from New Zealand and Denmark dropped out, and a Swedish rider collapsed after the finish and had to be hospitalized. The symptoms that these athletes developed undeniably indicated heat exhaustion. (See Table 3.1 on page 33.)

Research has proven that athletes involved in endurance sports other than distance cycling experience similar risks for overheating. In the 1970s, studies conducted by Dr. David Costill at the Human Performance Laboratory at Ball State University found that athletes who drank fluids during a two-hour run lowered their body temperatures by two degrees when compared with athletes who did not rehydrate. Without fluid intake, one athlete's temperature reached 105.5°F during exercise, but it only reached 103.6°F when he drank fluids. Body temperatures above 104.5°F cause great physical and mental stress and are extremely dangerous. Therefore, fluid replacement is absolutely critical during training or competition—especially on a hot day.

If you're preparing for competition, it's wise to drink extra fluids in the few days before you compete, because drinking ensures maximum tissue hydration at the start of an event. You should also drink fluids before and at frequent intervals during a long event, in order to keep your body temperature at safe levels.

Table 3.1. Symptoms of Overheating

BODY TEMPERATURE	SYMPTOMS
101–104°F	Muscle weakness
	Fatigue
104–105°F	Disorientation
	Severe muscle weakness
	Loss of balance
Above 105°F	Diminished sweating
	Loss of consciousness

Do Men Perspire More Than Women Do?

Some studies have suggested that women do not run as great a risk as men of becoming too dehydrated during exercise. The idea is that women sweat more efficiently than men and therefore lose less fluid. In a study to see if women really do have an edge in hot, humid weather, twelve runners—six female and six male— ran twenty-five miles in the hot Georgia sun. Temperatures during the run varied from 77 to 97 degrees, and relative humidity averaged a saunalike 70 to 80 percent.

These twelve volunteers were all in great shape. The men had been running an average of fifty-two miles per week, while the women had been averaging fifty-three miles per week. The men

continued

completed the twenty-five miles in an average of 173.5 minutes, while the women required about 183.8 minutes. Despite the time differences, all of the men and women were actually running at about 75 percent of maximum effort.

Just before they set out on their run, all twelve runners drank 14 ounces of a beverage containing carbohydrate and electrolytes. During the run, the men each drank approximately 29 ounces of fluid, while the women drank about 23 ounces each. Interestingly, sweat rates for the men turned out to be far higher. Men sweated out 1.70 liters of water per hour, and totaled about 3.80 liters during the run. Women, on the other hand, lost only about 1.25 liters each hour, totaling 2.65 liters of fluid. Thus, the average male runner lost about a liter more of water than the average female runner during the twenty-five-mile run. Women also finished the run with lower body temperatures, lost less blood-plasma volume, and maintained better levels of electrolytes in their blood.

This doesn't mean that women should be less concerned about replacing fluids when running on hot, humid days, however. The differences between the sexes weren't great enough to warrant totally different guidelines for women. In the heat, it's usually best to be on the safe side and drink plenty of fluids.

DEPLETION OF MUSCLE FUELS

During intense short-term exercise, fatigue can result from depletion of muscle glycogen. As explained in Chapter 2, this is because glucose is the only fuel source that your muscles use to generate energy through the anaerobic pathways, which last from ten seconds to several minutes in duration. During long-term exercise, the aerobic pathway kicks in for energy production. Fatty acids and amino acids are burned in addition to glucose as fuel for aerobic metabolism, providing a wider range of energy resources.

Studies have shown, however, that glycogen depletion contributes to muscle fatigue even during long-term exercise. When subjects exercised to exhaustion at 80 percent of their maximum capacity, the glycogen content of their muscles dropped to near zero in about ninety minutes. Endurance was increased when glycogen storage capacity in the muscles was enhanced through carbohydrate loading. (For a detailed discussion of carbohydrate loading, see Chapter 16.) This suggests that your muscles' initial glycogen content plays an important role in exercise performance. Because glycogen is a crucial fuel for energy production, your muscle cells attempt to conserve glycogen during extended exercise. As you continue to exercise, fat stores are mobilized and fatty acids are used in approximately equal amounts as glycogen to provide energy. Finally, protein begins to provide a greater percentage of energy.

If you exercise primarily to burn fat, you'll be happy to know that it's possible to train your muscles to become more efficient in using fat as a fuel source by completing several extended training sessions, each lasting more than two hours. This method stimulates the enzymes responsible for the conversion of stored fat into energy, which will enable you to burn a higher percentage of fat and conserve glycogen for more strenuous efforts. The increased capacity of trained athletes to use fat, and the tendency of their muscles to release more fatty acids from fat tissue, suggests that training can shift the proportion of energy produced through the metabolism of fat.

LOW BLOOD GLUCOSE

In addition to providing necessary energy for muscle contraction, glucose is a vital source of energy for the brain and nervous system. Although fatty acids and amino acids can be used for voluntary muscle movement, glucose is the only fuel that can be used in sufficient amounts for nervous system function. In fact, 50 to 60 percent of the glucose supplied by the liver is used strictly for brain and nervous system function.

During the early phase of exercise, most of the energy supplied by

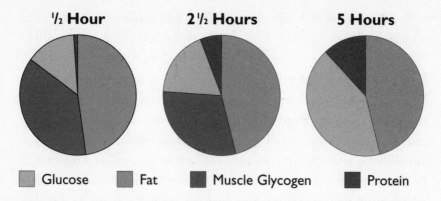

Figure 3.1. Proportions of fuel used during exercise. As exercise duration increases, your body relies less on muscle glycogen, and more on blood glucose, fat, and protein.

carbohydrate comes from muscle glycogen. As exercise continues and muscle glycogen stores run low, glycogen contributes less and less as a source of energy. Figure 3.1 above shows the proportions of nutrient fuels that are used during exercise. After about two hours of endurance exercise, muscle glycogen stores decrease rapidly. This reduced reliance on muscle glycogen is balanced by an increased reliance on blood glucose for fuel.

After two to three hours of exercise, the majority of carbohydrate energy appears to be derived from glucose, which is transported from circulating blood into the exercising muscles. This causes blood glucose to decline to relatively low levels. The liver, which has been supplying some amount of glucose from its glycogen stores, reduces its output due to depletion of liver glycogen. Fatigue occurs because there is not enough blood glucose available to compensate for the depleted muscle glycogen.

Studies by E. H. Christensen and O. Hansen in the 1960s demonstrated that subjects who exercised to exhaustion and then consumed 200 grams of glucose extended their performance by one hour. In this experiment, the nervous system's fuel had been depleted and restored. These results suggest that exhaustion may sometimes be a phenomenon of the central nervous system and not only the result of depleted muscle fuel stores.

As a long race continues, many athletes consume sports drinks, carbohydrate gels, and sports bars in an attempt to avoid fatigue. The use of these products helps athletes to keep blood glucose levels elevated to maintain central nervous system function, in addition to providing carbohydrate to working muscles. Research by Edward Coyle, Ph.D., from the University of Texas, has shown that during exercise, athletes are capable of absorbing up to 80 grams of carbohydrate per hour. This can delay fatigue by as much as thirty to sixty minutes, because the working muscles can rely primarily on blood glucose for energy.

INCREASED LACTIC-ACID LEVELS

Lactic acid is a byproduct of anaerobic metabolism when not enough oxygen is available to produce energy. Under most circumstances, lactic acid diffuses into your bloodstream to be transported to your heart, liver, and nonworking muscles, where it is converted back into glucose. As you begin to exercise harder, more lactic acid builds up in your muscles and must be removed by your blood. The lactic-acid level of your blood, therefore, continues to increase as exercise intensity increases. If this level of intensity is maintained, you will soon reach your lactate threshold, defined as the point at which the level of lactic acid in your blood is greater than your body can metabolize. Figure 3.2 on page 38 illustrates how blood-lactate concentration increases with an increase in exercise intensity.

Most coaches and scientists consider the lactate threshold to be an excellent indicator of an athlete's potential for endurance performance. The ability to exercise at a high intensity without accumulating lactic acid is very beneficial. Generally, in two athletes with similar oxygen uptakes, the athlete with the higher lactate threshold will perform better in endurance activities. Laboratory and field experiments suggest that training can increase the amount of lactic acid produced and tolerated by athletes. This adaptation probably results from an increased efficiency of aerobic

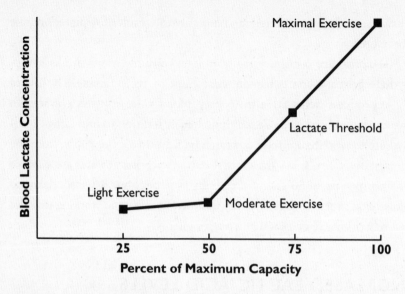

Figure 3.2. Blood lactate concentration during exercise. As exercise intensity increases, the lactic-acid level in the blood also increases.

metabolism as well as an increase in the number of capillaries that deliver oxygen to the muscles.

Lactic-acid buildup causes burning pain and muscle fatigue if it is not removed quickly from the muscles and metabolized by the body. Although lactic acid can be tolerated for short periods of time, you will need to back off the intensity to allow for adequate oxygen and blood flow to the muscles to help with removal and metabolism of the lactic acid. This allows your bloodstream to carry the lactic acid away and to supply your tissues with oxygen for aerobic metabolism.

Lactic Acid: Facts and Myths

Most exercisers recognize lactic acid as an enemy of high-intensity exertion and athletic performance. Carbohydrate along with fat and small amounts of protein provides energy to the cells of the body. It can be stored in muscles as glycogen or it can be obtained directly from the bloodstream as glucose. When either glycogen or glucose is broken down completely to provide energy, oxygen is needed for the process of aerobic metabolism to be complete.

When there is not enough oxygen available in active skeletal muscle cells, the process cannot be completed and lactic acid begins to appear in the exercising muscles. The lactic acid eventually moves out of the muscles, but several misconceptions exist about how and when it is removed.

The first myth is that lactic acid remains in the muscles for hours or even days after strenuous exercise. The fact is that lactic acid rapidly moves out of the muscle cells into the bloodstream and lactic acid levels in the muscles return to resting values in sixty minutes. Low-intensity aerobic exercise can actually speed up the process. After a hard effort or interval, light to moderate exercise will keep the blood flowing through the muscles, allowing the lactic acid to be removed from the system more rapidly and effectively.

The second myth is that lactic acid is related to *delayed onset muscle soreness* (DOMS), which may develop several hours or even days after particularly strenuous or unaccustomed exercise. It is not related, however, because the lactic acid has long ago moved out of the muscle. DOMS is likely to be caused by microscopic damage in muscle cells and by inflammation, not lactic-acid residue.

The third myth is that massage can rid the muscles of lactic acid. Massage feels good and has been shown to have therapeutic value; however, lactic acid is removed from the muscles by the circulatory system and from blood and fluid by the body's metabolic process. Again, the lactic acid is long gone by the time you reach the massage table.

The fourth myth is that lactic acid is the cause of fatigue during long-term exercise. It is not the cause but it is one of the causes. During high-intensity exercise lasting thirty seconds to several minutes, when adequate oxygen is not available, lactic acid does very temporarily cause the muscle to stop functioning properly to produce energy. In long-lasting aerobic exercise (two to four hours), muscle glycogen depletion (not lactic-acid buildup) causes the athlete to "hit the wall," or experience extreme muscle fatigue.

Now that you've been warned about a few of the lactic acid myths, here are some facts:

- The formation of lactic acid during intense exercise or sports competition is the probable cause of the uncomfortable burning sensation that occurs in muscles as fatigue sets in.
- The buildup of lactic acid during long-term exercise can be taken as an indication of poor aerobic (cardiovascular) fitness. When performing at the same exercise intensity, less lactic acid production means a better state of aerobic fitness.
- When large quantities of lactic acid have been produced in muscle cells, some of it can be utilized as energy by the muscle cell that produced it when oxygen becomes available during recovery. But most of the lactic acid will either be removed from the muscles by the circulatory system, be taken from the blood by other muscles and used for energy, or be carried to the liver and stored as glycogen.
- When performing high-intensity exercise to exhaustion, athletes generate higher lactic-acid levels than nonathletes. This can be related to enhanced anaerobic metabolism or, more probably, to an athlete's ability to continue to exercise longer than nonathletes despite great discomfort.

What Causes Muscle Cramps?

Perhaps the simplest way to describe a cramp is as an out-of-control muscle contraction that locks the muscle in a painful and sustained spasm. Unlike a normal muscle contraction, you have no control over when or where a cramp may strike—and if you don't act quickly, it can put you in a great deal of pain.

continued

The cause of cramps is elusive. Several theories exist, but the most common one is that cramps result from exercise-induced dehydration. When you exercise heavily, you can lose large quantities of water through perspiration. This water loss lowers blood volume, so there is less blood going to muscles to deliver oxygen, resulting in a muscle spasm. Another possible cause of cramps related to dehydration is electrolyte imbalance. The electrolytes sodium and potassium, together with calcium and magnesium, help regulate muscle relaxation and contraction. Because you may lose electrolytes through extreme sweating, dehydration can contribute to an electrolyte imbalance. If there's an imbalance of these nutrients, muscles may contract involuntarily.

Muscles that are overly fatigued or overworked are prone to cramps; thus, people who are not well trained are more likely to suffer from them. Some people are naturally more susceptible, and this may be due to inherently low electrolyte and mineral levels. Cold weather also seems to precipitate cramps in some athletes. Other less common causes include diabetes and circulatory and neurological disorders. Therefore, if you experience persistent cramps, you should consult your doctor.

Regardless of the cause, the treatment for immediate relief of muscle cramps is the same in every case: gently stretch the muscle as best you can. Also apply pressure to the muscle while stretching to help unlock the cramp. Gentle massage can also be beneficial. The importance of good warm-up and cool-down periods cannot be emphasized enough. Stretching thoroughly before and after your workout can stop cramps before they start. If painful muscle cramps habitually wake you up at night, also stretch before going to bed. Guidelines for stretching are presented in Chapter 18. Fortunately, there are several other steps that you can take to prevent cramps altogether.

continued

First, keep in mind the role of dehydration in causing cramps, and drink plenty of fluids to remain sufficiently hydrated, especially if you're exercising outdoors or in a hot and humid environment. Don't let thirst determine when you should drink fluids—by the time you're thirsty, you may already be 2 to 3 percent dehydrated. Because satisfying your thirst does not necessarily mean that you have satisfied your body's need for fluids, you should continue to replenish fluids, even if you think you're not thirsty. Chances are, your body is!

Also remember that it's crucial to get adequate amounts of nutrients such as sodium, potassium, calcium, and magnesium in your diet, because these minerals are responsible for proper muscle contraction and relaxation. Magnesium appears to be especially critical for triggering the relaxation of tensed muscles. However, simply popping a magnesium supplement is not the answer. In order to be most effective, magnesium needs to be properly balanced with calcium. A 2-to-1 ratio of magnesium to calcium is thought by many experts to provide the ideal balance of these important minerals for muscle relaxation. This ratio should not be confused with the 2-to-1 ratio of calcium to magnesium that is necessary for healthy bones. (See Chapter 14.) To help relieve muscle spasms and soreness, it is recommended that you supplement with 800 milligrams of magnesium and 400 milligrams of calcium daily.

Many athletes underestimate the effect that a change in environment can have on their ability to exercise. It's important that you acclimate slowly to weather changes. Take about two weeks to adjust to hot- or cold-weather temperature changes by gradually increasing the duration and intensity, and cut back slightly during seasonal transitions. This will allow your body to adjust with a minimal amount of physical stress. If you are vacationing in

continued

a dramatically different climate, take it easy on yourself for several days both while on holiday and when you arrive home.

Finally, consider the types of medication that you take. Various drugs such as diuretics and bronchial dilators have been implicated as causes of muscle cramps for some people. If you suffer from cramps and take any kind of medication, consult your physician to see if this may be the cause.

CENTRAL FATIGUE

In addition to focusing on the causes of muscle fatigue, recent research has also centered on mental fatigue during exercise. Mental fatigue is experienced physically. This is commonly called central fatigue because it results from impaired function of the central nervous system. Although central fatigue does not affect your muscles directly, it can reduce your capacity to perform.

Dr. Eric Newsholme of Oxford University has uncovered a correlation between levels of the amino acid tryptophan in the brain and the degree of mental fatigue. When tryptophan enters the brain, it can depress the central nervous system, causing sleepiness and the sensation of physical fatigue. Normally, there are sufficient amounts of the branched-chain amino acids (BCAAs) leucine, isoleucine, and valine in the blood to regulate the entry of tryptophan into the brain. During long-term exercise, however, muscle cells begin to use greater amounts of amino acids for energy. Your body prefers to use the BCAAs for energy because they can actually take the place of glucose in energy pathways. As your muscles begin to use the BCAAs for energy, the level of BCAAs drops, which allows for the entry of tryptophan into the brain, causing mental fatigue.

Research suggests that regular supplementation with BCAAs during long-term exercise can prevent or forestall central fatigue by preventing tryptophan from entering the brain. Supplementation before and during exercise has been proven to increase performance during a soccer game and after a thirty-kilometer race. Likewise, in a study of 193 marathoners, BCAA supplementation improved performance in the slower runners. Additional research is being conducted on this fascinating area of study. More will be presented on this subject in Chapter 6.

CONCLUSION

Today, sports scientists and nutritionists know that dehydration and carbohydrate depletion are not the only two factors that cause fatigue. Factors such as elevated lactic-acid levels and central fatigue also contribute to exhaustion. By making sure that you're properly hydrated before and during exercise, and by consuming enough of the nutrients that your body needs to fuel activity, you can greatly reduce your chances of hitting the wall.

Clearly, minimizing fatigue is one step toward maximizing performance. Rebuilding and repairing muscle tissue is another important factor in the strength and endurance equation. Before we can discuss how your muscles recover and develop after exercise, however, we have to look at the kinds of muscle damage that are caused by exercise. Just what are your muscles recovering from? Read on to find out.

4

What Causes Muscle Soreness?

There will be times when your muscles are stiff and sore the day after an intense training session no matter what your level of fitness or athletic skill is. You may wonder how your body could let you down like this, especially if you've already put so much time and effort into your exercise program. Whatever you did, you did too much. Now it's the day after and you have an athletic hangover. Despite the pain, you may choose to stick to your training schedule without decreasing intensity or duration. Perhaps you've taken to heart the "no pain, no gain" theory of training, and you actually find encouragement in your aching muscles. But what you and many other dedicated athletes don't know, and should be aware of, is that you're putting tremendous strain on your body—strain that could have long-term adverse effects on your physical and emotional health.

In the past, lactic-acid buildup was considered to be the cause of prolonged muscle fatigue and discomfort. However, lactic acid is completely washed out of the muscles within the sixty minutes after your exercise session. Since muscle soreness does not make itself known until twenty-four to thirty-six hours later, it's been necessary to seek out other explanations.

MECHANICAL DAMAGE

Current scientific research points to muscle damage as the primary cause of muscle soreness. When you strain your muscles, you produce localized damage such as microscopic tears to muscle fiber membranes and protein filaments. Over the twenty-four hours following strenuous exercise, the damaged muscles become swollen and sore. In addition, there is increased blood flow to the muscles, which causes the muscle tissues to swell. Muscle nerves perceive this abnormal state and send pain messages to your brain as soon as you try to move the morning after overexertion. By moving sore muscles, you increase circulation, which brings protein and other nutrients to muscles that need to be repaired. Moving stiff and sore muscles also helps to reduce swelling. This gradually begins to restore them to a normal state. However, you will not be able to exercise to your full potential because the damaged muscles have lost some strength.

Scientists have identified a biochemical marker called *creatine kinase* (CK) that is an excellent measure of muscle damage. CK is an enzyme used in metabolism that is found mainly in the cells of skeletal and heart muscle. When skeletal muscle is damaged due to a muscle tear or from overuse, CK begins to leak out of the muscles' cells, and blood levels of CK rise within the hour. Research suggests that the rise in CK is proportionate to the amount of skeletal muscle damage.

Typical short-term treatments for sore muscles include stretching, massage, topical application of sports balms or creams, submersion in a hot tub, or a session in the sauna. Some athletes also turn to aspirin, ibuprofen (Advil, Motrin), and other anti-inflammatory medication to reduce pain and inflammation. The real cure for muscle soreness, however, is prevention. The key is to gradually increase the difficulty and duration of your training program. Also, remember to stretch before and after every exercise session, and to warm up and cool down properly. You will find guidelines for stretching in Chapter 18.

Remember that aerobic activities, such as cycling, running, and swimming, and stop-and-go sports, such as basketball, use certain muscles that are not used regularly in daily life. The principle of *specificity of training* must be kept in mind: your muscles, tendons, and ligaments should be allowed to adapt to a particular sport, activity, or movement pattern over a period of time.

As we grow older, our muscles and their surrounding tissues lose elasticity, so we feel soreness and tightness more quickly than we did when we were in high school. Individuals who stay in shape into their thirties and forties should be able to exercise with minimal muscle soreness. After a very hard day of aerobic exercise or an intense session in the weight room, however, their muscles may feel somewhat stiff. Again, thorough warm-up and cool-down periods that include stretching should minimize this discomfort.

FREE-RADICAL DAMAGE

Recently, a great deal of research has focused on the link between free-radical formation and muscle damage. Free radicals are continuously formed as a normal consequence of body processes and are also caused by environmental factors such as air pollution and radiation. You may be surprised to find out, however, that exercise has been associated with the formation of free radicals as well. So what are these molecules, and how are they a threat to you, the health-conscious athlete?

All of your body's cells are made up of atoms that, in turn, contain paired particles called *electrons*. When every electron in an atom is paired with another electron, the atom is said to be stable. A free radical is an atom or molecule (group of atoms) that is short one electron and therefore is considered to be highly unstable. In order to restabilize itself, the free radical will actively seek out and steal an electron from another part of the cell. Free radicals are also known as *oxidants* because oxygen is usually the atom that loses an electron and then snatches other molecules' electrons. Therefore, free-radical damage is also known as *oxidative stress*.

There is evidence that long-term aerobic activity, including running, bicycling, and cross-country skiing, increases the production of these highly unstable molecules. Free radicals can damage muscle cell membranes and increase protein breakdown. They can also attack the walls of your muscle cells and mitochondria, and they are at least partially to blame for muscle inflammation and soreness, which contribute to reduced endurance.

Research has shown that antioxidants may be vital components in reducing post-exercise muscle soreness. Antioxidants are vitamins and vitaminlike nutrients that can neutralize free radicals. Vitamins E and C are some of the better known antioxidants. These two nutrients are discussed individually in Chapter 8.

THE CORTISOL RESPONSE

Cortisol is a hormone that is released in response to all kinds of stress, including psychological, physical, and emotional stresses. Exercise places physical stress on your body, which stimulates the release of cortisol from small glands called *adrenal glands* attached to the top of each kidney. The primary role of cortisol is to help mobilize energy for the body. It does this by attacking muscle tissue directly and increasing the rate at which protein in the muscles is broken down. In addition to this, cortisol impedes the entry of amino acids into muscle cells for protein synthesis, and instead helps to transport them to the liver to be used for energy. This is why individuals involved in strength training may experience a decrease in muscle mass if they do not take the necessary steps to reduce the release of cortisol and to rebuild muscle protein.

For a number of years, athletes have used anabolic (muscle-building) steroids, which negate the effects of cortisol by helping the body to build itself back up. With steroid use, amino acids are taken up by the muscles at a higher rate to help repair some of the damage caused by cortisol when it extracts important nutrients for energy. However, the long-term use of anabolic steroids has been linked to the development of illnesses such as liver cancer and heart disease. In Chapter 10, we'll see how the R^4 system can help you blunt the rise of cortisol naturally.

Can Sports Creams and Anti-inflammatory Drugs Blitz Post-Exercise Pain?

Stand in any locker room and chances are you will smell the aroma of menthol. The source of the scent is a tube of one of the dozens of products on the market that have become a part of post-exercise pain relief. Technically known as analgesics or counterirritants, they come in ointment or cream form or as a liniment. Their use in sports is strictly to aid in "warm-up" or as a source of relief for muscle soreness.

They are known as counterirritants because they produce a slight irritation of the skin and therefore create a sensation of warmth ranging from mild to intense. However, there is more actual buildup of heat from the rubbing of the cream into the muscles than that caused by the counterirritants. In other words, the heat that builds up in the muscles as a result of the massaging action is greater than that caused by the use of the analgesic itself.

The most popular ingredient in analgesics is methyl salicylate, found in wintergreen oil or prepared synthetically. When put on your skin, it causes the skin to turn red and produces a feeling of warmth. Methyl salicylate is safe when used no more than three or four times per day. But someone who is sensitive to aspirin should monitor the use of methyl salicylate since it is related to aspirin.

Menthol is the second most widely used ingredient in these

continued

products and is produced synthetically or extracted from pepper-mint oil. Menthol stimulates the nerves that perceive cold while depressing those that perceive pain. The immediate effect is a sense of coolness, followed by sensations of warmth.

With this combination of menthol and methyl salicylate, a mixed sensation of coolness and warmth is sent to the brain, which diminishes the perception of pain. This is why these prod-ucts are used after a hard effort when you experience soreness in your muscles. The fragrance of the menthol also acts psychologi-cally to take your mind off your sore muscles.

Never apply these products to bruised or abraded skin, since absorption into the body can produce unwanted effects. If a rash develops, stop using the product and try a different one. Finally, avoid using counterirritants near sensitive areas, such as lips, eyes, and crotch.

Balms with counterirritant ingredients like camphor or men-thol function by stimulating the skin to divert attention from muscle soreness. They usually produce warmth or a tingling sen-sation when applied, but because they contain no active ingredi-ents, they don't really have any effect on the muscles under the surface.

Aspirin or other anti-inflammatory medications should not be used to help relieve soreness. If microtrauma or acute injury is present, aspirin will increase blood flow and swelling to the area. These medications will also inhibit the release of prostaglandins, hormones that may be important in muscle repair. This can delay healing.

CAUSES OF DELAYED ONSET MUSCLE SORENESS (DOMS)

While many people experience just acute muscle soreness, there are many individuals who experience muscle soreness that does not begin until several hours after exercise and lingers on for a day or two after exercise. Much of what causes acute muscle soreness is still the villain in the days after a hard workout. The soreness felt in the twenty-four to forty-eight hours after a workout, often referred to as delayed onset muscle soreness (DOMS), appears to be caused by the continued disruption or damage to the muscle fibers. It has also been suggested that soreness is caused by the stimulation of free nerve endings around the muscle fibers, which are receptors for the noxious stimuli associated with muscle damage. Finally, soreness that continues to progress over several days could be due to the continued production of free radicals and white blood cells coming into the damaged area due to inflammation and destroying of muscle proteins. Thus, much of the soreness appears to be damage related. However, investigators have also made measurements of intramuscular fluid pressure and found it to be elevated after exercise, which resulted in soreness but was not necessarily related to damage. So the causes of DOMS are not necessarily restricted to damage of muscle fibers.

The first thing you should know is that nonsteroidal anti-inflammatory drugs (NSAIDs) such as ibuprofen and acetaminophen do not work on DOMS, and will actually interfere with muscle recuperation. A study published in the *American Journal of Physiology* demonstrates this in a striking way. Researchers gave twenty-four men recommended doses of ibuprofen, acetaminophen, or a placebo (a "dummy pill" that doesn't contain active ingredients) on the day following a hardcore eccentric weight workout. They then measured both muscle soreness and *skeletal muscle fractional synthesis rate* (SMFSR)—the muscle-building response to exercise twenty-four hours after the workout. They found that not only did NSAIDs not help with muscle soreness at all, they completely halted all SMFSR (that is, the muscle made no gains toward recovery). While the placebo group increased its SMFSR by 76 percent, there was no increase in the NSAID groups. In other words, muscle building was completely negated by the NSAIDs.

On the brighter side, as we will see in subsequent chapters, nutritional and nonnutritional approaches can be undertaken in the hours after training or competition to greatly reduce the incidence of DOMS. Proper intake of carbohydrate, protein, and antioxidants and the use of stretching and massage will greatly reduce the incidence of DOMS in your training program.

CONCLUSION

Sore muscles are usually damaged muscles. As with any injury, sore muscles must be given time to heal. Keep in mind that the majority of muscle development occurs during the post-exercise recovery period. When you disregard pain and stiffness, or use too many NSAIDs, you are actually doing more harm than good because you are not giving your body time to recover from the mechanical and biochemical damage caused by exercise. And getting right back on the treadmill, so to speak, will only cause further damage to muscles that have already been weakened. These effects, coupled with physical discomfort, will make it impossible for you to exercise at peak capacity during subsequent training sessions.

Many athletes erroneously believe that extended muscle soreness is caused by a buildup of lactic acid that can be mitigated by warming down after a run. Although lactic acid is often responsible for soreness felt during and right after running, research has shown that next-day soreness has other causes and should be handled differently.

Fortunately, research has proven that recovery can negate some of the physical effects of exercise. Chapter 5 examines the three critical phases of recovery during which energy stores are replenished and muscle damage is repaired. In doing so, it establishes the foundation for the R^4 System for Peak Performance.

Recovery: Your Key to Peak Performance

Your ability to continue exercising or competing day after day is limited by how quickly your muscles recover after exertion. Recovery means that your body returns to a normal, balanced state through the restoration of body fluids, replenishment of energy stores, and repair of damaged muscle tissues. In addition, your immune system, which is compromised by strenuous exercise, can be enhanced with adequate rest and careful attention to nutrition. By taking the proper steps to aid your body's recovery from exercise, you will increase your level of performance during training sessions or competitive events. More important, your overall health and strength will be improved.

THE THREE PHASES OF RECOVERY

Recovery from extended exercise is a complex process, but it can be broken down into three parts. The first phase of recovery, known as the rapid phase, occurs in the first thirty minutes after exercise. This is followed by the intermediate phase, which lasts up to two hours. The longer phase of recovery occurs during the remaining twenty hours before your next exercise session.

The Rapid Phase

The rapid phase of recovery begins when you finish your training session and lasts for approximately thirty minutes. During this time, your body's metabolic rate slows and begins to return to pre-exercise levels. Your heart rate, respiratory rate, and body temperature start to return to their lower resting levels. Blood levels of certain hormones, such as cortisol and testosterone, which were elevated during exercise, begin to decrease. At the same time, your muscles start to replenish their stores of creatine phosphate and ATP, which were depleted to fuel activity. This is also the period during which your body removes excess lactic acid that may have accumulated in your muscles. The majority of the lactic acid enters the bloodstream and circulates to the liver and inactive muscles, where it is reconverted into glucose.

The metabolic and physiological processes that occur during the rapid phase of recovery can be hastened by gentle exercise during the cooldown period. Exercising at 40 to 60 percent of maximum effort for five to ten minutes helps to keep your blood circulating at an increased rate. Keeping blood flow at a higher-than-normal rate during this phase aids in the removal of lactic acid from your muscles and rapidly transports it to the appropriate sites for conversion to glucose.

The Intermediate Phase

The intermediate phase of recovery continues in the ninety minutes to two hours after exercise. During this time, your body begins the process of restoring fluid volumes, called rehydration. This is also the most critical period for the replenishment of muscle glycogen, in which the hormone insulin plays a vital role. Insulin facilitates the transport of

glucose from your blood into your muscle cells. It also stimulates glycogen synthase, an enzyme in your muscle cells that is responsible for converting glucose into glycogen for storage.

Research conducted by Dr. John Ivy at the University of Texas at
Austin's Exercise Physiology and Metabolism Laboratory has provided
insight into why the intermediate phase is such a critical stage in the recovery process. Dr. Ivy discovered that muscle cells are most sensitive to
insulin during this time. This means that when a sufficient source of carbohydrate is present, glycogen replenishment occurs at a faster rate. In
fact, the speed of glycogen synthesis in the two hours following exercise
is almost two to three times faster than normal.

In order to take full advantage of this increased insulin sensitivity, Dr.
Ivy recommends drinking a carbohydrate-containing beverage such as a
sports drink as soon after an event or training session as possible. If you
don't consume a carbohydrate supplement during this period, you'll miss
the period of maximum insulin sensitivity, and the rate of glycogen recovery will be significantly slowed. Thus, the longer you wait to replenish
your glycogen stores, the longer it will take you to recover. As you will see
in Chapter 7, consuming the proper ratio of carbohydrate and protein in
your post-exercise meal or snack can increase your body's sensitivity to
insulin during this critical phase as well.

The Longer Phase

The longer phase of recovery spans the two to twenty hours following
a workout. Carbohydrate replenishment continues in this interval, although at a lesser rate than during the first two hours following exercise.
It's recommended that you consume 3 to 5 grams of carbohydrate per
pound of your body weight over a twenty-four hour period of recovery.
Most of your carbohydrate intake during this time should come from foods
such as pasta, breads, and vegetables. These are complex carbohydrates,
which consist of long chains of glucose that must first be broken down during digestion. This breakdown ensures a slow, steady supply of glycogen.

A crucial element in the long-term recovery process is muscle repair.

During heavy exercise, the membranes of muscle fibers, the connective tissue surrounding them, and the actin and myosin filaments of your muscles are damaged. Less strenuous exercise also damages muscles, but to a lesser degree. Therefore, whether you engage in a moderate activity, such as jogging, or a more strenuous exercise like weightlifting, sprinting, or high-intensity running or cycling, your muscles require time and nutrients for repair. The long-term phase of recovery is the period in which muscles are repaired and adapt to exercise, which increases strength and endurance. The question, then, concerns how much "damage" you must do in order for your muscles to become stronger. Do you have to exercise to the point of muscle soreness?

"That's probably not necessary, because you can go in small steps and get the same types of changes," says William Evans, Ph.D., of the Nutrition, Metabolism, and Exercise Laboratory at the University of Arkansas for Medical Sciences in Little Rock. In fact, when you have extreme soreness and pain—the kind that gives you trouble jogging, moving your limbs, or lifting a heavy object—research shows that your strength is reduced, sometimes by as much as 25 percent. And the more you hurt, the longer it takes to recover your strength so that you can again exercise at your peak capacity.

The stresses of exercise also compromise your immune system, making you more susceptible to colds and infections. The intensity of your chosen activity, as well as your physical condition, influences the impact that exercise will have on your immune system, according to Dr. Evans. But, as you will see in Chapter 8, this damage can be minimized or even prevented.

ALCOHOL AND RECOVERY

After a tough workout, some individuals like to kick back with a few beers. But will the alcohol slow recovery? I certainly don't recommend drinking beer after a hard workout, but I know that you'll probably drink it anyway if you are accustomed to doing so.

In some sports, but notably team sports, the tradition is to "celebrate" the outcome by drinking alcohol together. This is often undertaken when the athlete is dehydrated and hasn't eaten for a number of hours, thus potentiating the absorption and effects of the alcohol. Often good sense goes out the window after a couple of drinks, and in a spirit of camaraderie or even competition, the athlete may overindulge considerably.

Just remember that alcohol slows your recovery by delaying rehydration and preventing carbohydrate from getting to your muscles. Alcohol is actually a diuretic. That said, you can have a couple of beers if you drink intelligently. First, drink a bottle or two of a recovery sports drink (see Chapter 10 for information on recovery sports drinks) until you're hydrated (your urine will be pale yellow to clear). Don't even think about having a beer until you've urinated at least once after your workout. Then, have your beer, along with a high-carbohydrate food. Alternate your beer with water or a sports drink, and stop at two unless you're prepared to skip your workout the next day.

Here are some guidelines for moderate alcohol intake after exercise:

- Rehydrate and refuel as a first priority after intense exercise.
- Remember that alcoholic drinks (more than 4 percent alcohol) are not ideal rehydration beverages. Nor do they provide a significant source of carbohydrate. These "myths" are often used as a rationalization to approve or excuse the heavy alcohol intake of some athletes.
- Once fluid and carbohydrate needs have been met, alcohol may be consumed in moderation.
- The vasodilation, or flushing of the skin with blood, caused by alcohol may increase heat loss in cold environments (for example, in winter sports). Take care to stay warm in such environments.

The Dangers of Overtraining

In *Lore of Running*, Dr. Timothy Noakes gives examples of several nationally ranked athletes who exhibited symptoms of overtraining syndrome (OTS). One athlete complained that he was lethargic and sleeping poorly. He also had less enthusiasm for training, and particularly for competition. He expressed concern that his legs felt "sore" and "heavy" and that the feelings had lasted for several training sessions. This athlete was obviously in need of complete rest from hard training.

The phenomena of overtraining are very real for the aerobic athlete. In training, it is a difficult but essential task to find your optimal training threshold and to not exceed the limits of your stress and adaptation capacities. Specific physiological and psychological changes are related to overtraining, which lead to a corresponding deterioration of athletic performance.

The symptoms of overtraining may be seen in an athlete who is eager to excel and begins to train frequently and intensely. At first, the athlete improves. After a while, however, his times stagnate and remain below his set goals. Anxious to pass the plateau, the athlete begins to train even harder. Instead of improving, his performance deteriorates and a sense of inadequacy and frustration develops. In addition to a decline in performance, there are corresponding changes in personality and behavior. The athlete gradually loses self-confidence and suffers from chronic fatigue.

Are you worried that you or someone you know is overtraining? It's important to watch out for the following symptoms:

Physical Changes
- Constipation or diarrhea
- Fatigue

continued

- Flu-like symptoms, including fever, chill, and aches
- Gradual weight loss
- Heavy feeling in legs
- Inability to complete training
- Increased morning heart rate
- Lack of appetite
- Muscle soreness
- Swelling in lymph nodes

Emotional and Behavioral Changes
- Anxiety
- Depression
- Desire to quit training
- Inability to concentrate
- Irritability
- Loss of enthusiasm for training and competition
- Sleep disturbances

In the early 1980s, Dick Brown, then administrator and physiologist for the world-class running club Athletics West, conducted an experiment to try to identify warning signs of overtraining. He asked athletes to record several indicators in their training diaries, including morning body weight, morning heart rate, and amount of sleep. His research showed that if an athlete's morning heart rate is at least 10 percent higher than normal, if the athlete receives 10 percent less sleep than usual, or if the athlete's weight is down 3 percent or more, the athlete's body has not recovered from the previous hard workout. Therefore, to be on the safe side, you should cut back on your workout if you are abnormal in two indicators. Abnormal readings for all three indicators are a red flag, signaling that you should take the day off.

In order to ensure that you prevent the complications of over-

continued

training before they occur, you should take the following measures into account:

- Use the nutritional principles of the R^4 System to make sure that you are maximizing recovery. These four principles are detailed in Part II.
- Sleep at least eight hours a night when you are engaged in a strenuous training program.
- Follow the guidelines presented in Part III to ensure that you are eating a balanced diet.
- Conduct at least eight weeks of endurance work to build up a good base of conditioning.
- Gradually build up the quantity and quality of training, so that you are prepared both physically and mentally for an increased volume of training. Do not increase the frequency, duration, or intensity of training sessions too quickly.
- Try to nap for fifteen minutes to a half-hour before an afternoon workout.
- Make sure that the intensity of your training is individualized to your level of fitness and experience.
- Use a training diary to record morning pulse rate, morning body weight, sleep patterns, medical problems, and training difficulties.

Remember that rest and recovery are essential if you want your muscles to grow and develop. The use of rest days on a periodic basis will increase your strength and allow you to perform at your peak level when you do exercise.

CONCLUSION

Once strenuous training or competition has ended for the day, sufficient rest and careful nutritional management become essential for future performance. Recovery begins the moment that you cross the finish line, walk in from the field, or get down off your bike. During the post-exercise period, your muscles must receive essential nutrients to recover from mechanical damage in the form of swelling and microscopic tears, oxidative damage caused by unstable free radicals, and tissue degradation due to the release of cortisol in response to exercise stress.

In these first few chapters, we have reviewed the physical structure of skeletal muscles and how they function to generate movement. You have also learned about the biochemistry behind muscle function—namely, the anaerobic and aerobic pathways in which the nutrient fuels (carbohydrate, fat, and protein) are used to generate energy for movement. And now that you know the story behind why athletes experience muscle fatigue and soreness, and how the human body is equipped to recover, we are ready to move on to the specifics of the R^4 System. Part II examines, in detail, the steps that you should take in order to optimize your recovery.

Part II

The R⁴ System for Peak Performance

In the past, you may have experienced days when you simply couldn't meet your training goals, no matter how hard you pushed yourself. Whether you were still aching from your previous workout, thwarted by a muscle cramp, or just plain exhausted, you simply weren't able to exercise at peak capacity. In such cases, what was your remedy for muscle soreness and fatigue? Did you take a day off from training, try painkillers, or use sports balms? Believe it or not, exercise-induced fatigue and soreness are not entirely inevitable. The truth is that you can, to some extent, avoid these unpleasant consequences.

Part II will guide you in maximizing your recovery with targeted nutrition. Each of the principles of the R⁴ System is discussed individually, so that you can learn how to refuel and rehydrate muscles during exercise, replenish glycogen after exercise, reduce muscle stress, and rebuild muscle protein. By following the simple guidelines outlined in the next few chapters, you'll be able to extend your endurance and increase your muscle strength within days, in addition to minimizing muscle pain and boosting immunity. All of these benefits will enable you to perform at a higher level than you've ever thought possible.

We will start off Part II with some guidelines on how to stay properly hydrated and fueled during long-term exercise. New research shows that you can reduce recovery time by maintaining proper nutrition and hydration during exercise.

6

Refuel and Rehydrate Muscles During Exercise

Over the past twenty years, many sports have seen major advances in athletic training. We now have an impressive array of tools to help athletes optimize their performance. Yet one tool that is still not fully utilized is muscle hydration and nutrition during exercise. It is an area that is often surrounded by misconceptions and inaccurate information. Proper hydration and nutrition is as integral to optimizing performance as are fitness and technique. Cutting-edge research coming out of leading exercise physiology laboratories in the past two decades has dramatically reshaped our views of how nutrition can improve muscle performance.

This chapter deals with the energy and fluid needs of muscles both during and after exercise. It also reviews some exciting research on how carbohydrate replenishment during exercise can blunt the effect of cortisol—a catabolic hormone released during exercise that breaks down muscle protein. You may already be familiar with some of this information, but you may find much of it surprising.

Muscle refueling has two components—fluid and energy. Both are essential. The benefits of replenishing energy and fluid during intense exercise include delay of fatigue, reduction in post-exercise muscle damage, improvement in endurance, and even a decrease in the stress hormone cortisol, which can break down muscle protein.

Sports drinks are undergoing a renaissance. Several years ago, the idea of combining carbohydrate with protein in an optimal ratio was born. It has been gaining in popularity among endurance athletes ever since. This trend is a result of the growing body of data documenting the synergism of protein/carbohydrate mixtures. Protein-containing sports drinks are, indeed, a major breakthrough in the ability of sports drinks to enhance performance.

FLUID AND ELECTROLYTE REPLACEMENT

Most athletes understand the relationship between exercise and water loss. Sweat is the body's coolant. During an intense workout, your muscles generate heat, which is carried by your blood through capillaries near the surface of your skin. Your sweat glands release sweat (made up of water and electrolyte minerals), which evaporates, cooling the skin and the blood just underneath. Cooled blood then flows back to cool your body's core.

Sweating is therefore an essential mechanism for regulating body temperature. However, the loss of water that comes with perspiration limits the capacity of your blood to carry vital nutrients, such as glucose, fatty acids, and oxygen, to working muscles. The capacity of the blood to remove the byproducts of metabolism, including carbon dioxide and lactic acid, is compromised as well. The result is an increased demand on the circulatory system, which is approximately 70 percent water.

The real issue is what happens during an intense workout or competition. Temperature, which is normally 98.6°F, may increase to 104°F. An elevation in body temperature above 104.5°F causes an increased demand on the cardiovascular system. Obviously, the key is to consume fluids before, during, and after a workout. Unfortunately, the human body is not well equipped to replenish the fluids that are lost through sweating and evaporation. We simply lack the capacity to take in and retain fluids at the rate they are lost during heavy exercise. This phenomenon is known as *involuntary dehydration*. The good news is that, by paying careful attention to what you drink and when you drink it, you can minimize dehydration and restore electrolyte, or salt, losses.

In order to understand how your body replenishes lost fluids, you should first understand what causes thirst. The thirst drive is dependent upon two factors: your body's blood volume and the concentration of salts, or electrolytes, in your blood. When you lose fluids during exercise through sweating, your blood volume decreases. This results in a corresponding increase in the concentration of electrolytes in your blood, which stimulates thirst.

Recent research has shown that your body absorbs more fluid when electrolytes such as sodium are added to water. In one study, six volunteers underwent two exposures to heat and then engaged in an exercise program that caused mild dehydration, resulting in a 2 to 3 percent decrease in body weight. Each volunteer then drank either water or a water and sodium solution to replenish fluids. During the three-hour rehydration period, subjects who drank water alone restored 68 percent of the fluid they lost, while subjects who drank the sodium solution replaced 82 percent of their lost fluids. What caused this marked difference? The addition of sodium to water helped to maintain the salt-dependent factor of the thirst drive, prompting the volunteers to continue drinking. This led to a more complete restoration of body fluids within the three-hour recovery period.

Electrolyte Replacement

Electrolytes such as sodium, chloride, potassium, and magnesium are necessary elements for muscle contraction and relaxation. In addition, electrolytes help maintain your body's fluid balance. During exercise, your body loses some amount of these minerals with water through sweating. Because electrolytes are found in blood plasma and muscle tissues in varying concentrations, measured in milliequivalents per liter (mEq/L), the concentrations lost through sweat vary as well. (See Table 6.1 below.)

Table 6.1. Electrolyte Concentrations in Blood Plasma, Muscle Tissue, and Sweat

	SODIUM (MEQ/L)	CHLORIDE (MEQ/L)	POTASSIUM (MEQ/L)	MAGNESIUM (MEQ/L)
BLOOD PLASMA	140	100	4	1.5
MUSCLE TISSUE	9	5	160	30
SWEAT	40–60	30–50	4–5	1.5–5.0

Whereas drinking pure water to quench your thirst quickly reduces the drive for additional fluid consumption, the addition of electrolytes leads to a more complete restoration of body water content. This is because electrolytes are salts, so they help maintain the salt-dependent element of thirst. This leads to more effective rehydration and regulation of your body temperature and cardiovascular function. Figure 6.1 on page 69 summarizes this principle.

SODIUM AND CHLORIDE

Sodium and chloride are electrolytes that help maintain the volume and balance of all the fluids outside your body's cells, such as blood. Sodium plays a particularly important role because it helps transport nutrients into cells so they can be used for energy production as well as tissue growth and repair. In addition, sodium functions in muscle contraction and nerve-impulse transmission.

The concentration of sodium and chloride lost in sweat is about one-third the concentration found in the plasma of your blood. Therefore, if you lose 9 pounds of sweat during a long race or training session, the electrolyte losses would be roughly 5 to 6 percent of your body's total sodium and chloride content.

Sodium and chloride are found in most foods and can be easily ob-

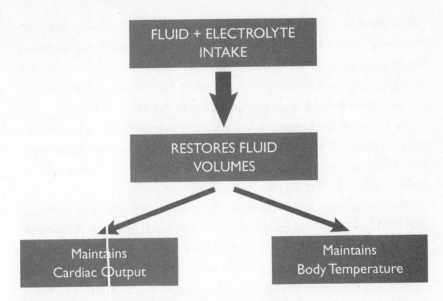

Figure 6.1. Restoration of fluid and electrolytes

tained through a balanced diet. Therefore, sodium or chloride deficiency generally occurs because of severe dehydration during long periods of exercise without proper fluid or electrolyte replenishment. The side effects include reduced performance, dizziness, and fainting.

POTASSIUM

Potassium is necessary for nerve transmission, muscle contraction, and glycogen formation. It also aids in maintaining cardiovascular system function. Whereas sodium and chloride are highly concentrated in the fluids outside of your cells, the concentration of potassium in the fluid within your cells is almost forty times greater than the concentration in your blood. Therefore, potassium losses through sweat are not nearly as great as sodium and chloride losses. It has been suggested, however, that this small percentage is enough to cause muscles to contract involuntarily, resulting in painful cramps that can stop you in your tracks. In addition, potassium losses can lead to heat intolerance.

Potassium is lost in a number of ways during and after exercise. Because potassium is stored together with glycogen in the muscle fibers, the breakdown of glycogen to supply energy to your muscles leads to an increased loss of potassium from the muscle cells. This results in a corresponding increase in the potassium concentration of your blood. After exercise, potassium is excreted in greater quantities in the urine.

To replenish the potassium loss resulting from exercise, try drinking a recovery sports drink that contains potassium. It's also wise to eat a balanced diet that includes foods high in potassium, such as dairy foods, bananas, oranges, kiwi fruit, potatoes, and tomato juice.

Because potassium is present in most foods, deficiency is rarely reported. Depletion is generally due to severe dehydration. A common cause of potassium depletion is prolonged use of diuretics, which promote potassium excretion by the kidneys. The symptoms of potassium deficiency are numerous, and include nausea, diminished reflex function, fluctuations in heartbeat, drowsiness, and muscular fatigue and weakness.

MAGNESIUM

Magnesium is found in all of your body's cells, although it is primarily located in the bones, muscles, and soft tissues. It's a necessary element in more than 300 enzyme reactions involving nerve transmission, muscle contraction, and especially ATP production.

Research has shown that increased physical activity can deplete the body's magnesium stores. In one study, twenty-six runners were found to have significantly lower levels of magnesium in their blood and urine after they completed a marathon. This could be because the body uses more magnesium during prolonged, intense exercise. When magnesium levels fall below a critical point, performance suffers, and athletes run a greater risk of developing muscle cramps.

Low blood-magnesium levels during exercise have also been cited as causes of muscle fatigue and irregular heartbeat. Magnesium deficiency can lead to dizziness, muscle weakness, irritability, and depression. Based on this information, it's important to consume a sports drink that contains magnesium in order to replenish what is lost during exercise. Sufficient magnesium can also be obtained by eating a balanced diet including magnesium-rich foods such as apples, avocados, bananas, brown rice, dairy foods, garlic, green leafy vegetables, soybeans, and whole grains.

Several studies have shown that supplementing the diet with moderate amounts of magnesium is not only beneficial in avoiding depletion, but may also improve endurance and strength. In a study of untrained subjects ranging from eighteen to twenty years of age who underwent a seven-week training schedule, greater improvements in muscle strength were found among those who took 560 milligrams of magnesium daily compared with those who received a placebo.

Hyponatremia

Jim was in good shape. He'd been cycling 200 miles a week in preparation for an upcoming 100-mile bike ride. One day, he decided to go on a long training ride alone, despite the ninety-degree heat. For the first forty miles he felt strong, so he decided to do another twenty-five miles. He drank a little of a sports drink designed to restore normal blood levels of electrolytes, but he relied mostly on water.

During the last twenty-five miles, hyponatremia—a relatively rare but potentially fatal condition in which blood levels of sodium sink dangerously low—came on rapidly. He finished the ride very slowly and began to vomit. Fortunately, he was able to make it to a hospital, where he had a seizure.

Full-blown cases of hyponatremia (sometimes called water intoxication) are relatively rare, striking roughly 0.1 to 4 percent of people who sweat steadily for hours in grueling long-distance events. The incidence of hyponatremia appears to be highest in events lasting more than four hours, especially at high tempera-

continued

tures and humidity. But the prevalence of warning symptoms is much higher; up to 25 percent of athletes seek attention in a medical tent during a long race.

Typically, conscientious athletes get in trouble because they adhere too diligently to one recommendation: the need to drink lots of fluids. They tend to ignore another recommendation: the need to keep electrolytes up. Indeed, for most endurance athletes, the real problem is drinking too much water, not failing to take in enough sodium.

If you drink only water, the sodium level in your blood becomes diluted. Normally, sodium is plentiful in the blood and relatively low inside cells. But when the concentration in the blood becomes too low compared with the amount inside cells—either because a person drank too much water, took in too little sodium, or both—water rushes into cells. The result is dangerous swelling, particularly in the brain, which can lead to brain damage, coma, and death.

Curiously, hyponatremia can strike whether a person is dehydrated, normally hydrated, or overhydrated because any of those conditions can occur while blood levels of sodium are too low. Further complicating things is that the symptoms of hyponatremia can be easily confused with those of heatstroke and heat exhaustion. With heat exhaustion, people feel ill, get nauseous, have muscle cramps, and may feel dizzy standing up quickly. With heatstroke, people have all those symptoms plus one more: mental-status changes—that is, there is confusion about who and where they are and what day it is. People with genuine heatstroke also typically have extremely high body temperatures. With hyponatremia, people also feel very ill and may have mental-status changes, but they don't have the high body temperatures associated with heatstroke. They also vomit forcefully and repeatedly

continued

and, unlike those with heat exhaustion, do not feel better by resting and cooling off. Some may have seizures.

Treatment of hyponatremia involves taking in fluid with sports
drinks when possible and promoting urine production, but some
people also need intravenous saline with a high concentration of
salt until blood electrolytes return to normal. If hyponatremia is
suspected, it is important to seek medical attention.

To protect yourself against hyponatremia, start by paying attention to how much you sweat. Individuals also vary considerably in how much sodium they lose in sweat. You may be a heavy
sodium loser if your sweat burns your eyes, tastes salty, or leaves a
white residue on your skin. You can also make sure you're getting
enough sodium by drinking sports drinks instead of plain water
during long events.

Fluid Consumption Guidelines

You should try to fully replace fluid and electrolyte losses that occur
during exercise. However, it is seldom possible to achieve this ideal of
complete compensation. Research has shown that most athletes are unable to tolerate drinking fluids at a rate exceeding 80 percent of the rate
of fluid loss during very high-intensity exercise in a hot environment. If
one loses 1.5 liters per hour in sweat, they can only hope to replace 1.2
liters in that hour. The upper limit of gastric emptying is about 0.6 to 1.2
liters per hour. (Gastric emptying is the rate at which your stomach contents are emptied into the intestines.) When too much fluid is consumed,
bloating and nausea can result. As a general rule, then, one should consume as much fluid as they can tolerate during workouts and competitions. The key is to drink fluids more often in smaller amounts. One can
often increase tolerance for fluid consumption during exercise simply by
practicing it consistently.

Different people lose fluids at different rates during exercise. Athletes can estimate their own standard rate of sweat loss by weighing themselves immediately before and after a typical workout. For example, suppose you lose 2 kilograms (4.4 pounds) during a sixty-minute workout. One kilogram translates to roughly one liter of fluid, or about 34 ounces. You should try to replace one liter of fluid for each hour of exercise. Note that higher environmental temperatures and higher exercise intensities increase the rate of fluid loss. Thus, in hot weather and at high-intensity levels, it is particularly important that you consume as much fluid as you can tolerate. In fact, many athletes use a CamelBak–type back-mounted hydration system in order to carry enough fluids during long training sessions to ensure adequate fluid replacement.

Again, water is not sufficient, because drinking water does not replace electrolyte losses that occur through perspiration. Rates of electrolyte loss also vary from one individual to the next, but in general, it is easier to fully compensate for electrolyte losses during exercise than for fluid losses. Most sports drinks are formulated to provide electrolytes and fluid in the proper ratio to make up for the effects of perspiration. A well-formulated sports drink should contain about 15 milligrams of sodium per ounce and about 5 milligrams of potassium per ounce.

For maximum effectiveness, you should consume several ounces of sports drink every fifteen minutes rather than taking in smaller amounts more frequently by sipping often. Consuming the drink at a cool temperature also results in faster gastric emptying and is therefore also advised. Table 6.2 on page 75 provides guidelines on suggested fluid intake versus sweat rate per hour.

Research has shown that most individuals' stomachs can empty only about 6 to 10 ounces of fluid every fifteen minutes during exercise. Amounts greater than that will just slosh around in your stomach. Some people process more or less than this, so experiment with how much your stomach will tolerate. If you have a hard time remembering to drink, use an alarm wristwatch or some other method to remind you it's time to drink.

Your sweat rate equals your pre-exercise weight minus your post-exercise weight, plus the amount of fluid consumed during exercise. Determine your typical "fluid shortfall" during exercise by measuring your

Table 6.2. Matching Fluid Intake with Sweat Loss

SWEAT RATE (POUNDS PER HOUR)	FLUID INTAKE (OUNCES)	FREQUENCY (MINUTES)
0.5	2	15
1.1	4	15
1.7	6.5	15
2.2	8.5	15
2.8	7	10
3.3	8.5	10
3.9	10	10

body weight before and after practices and competitions, with your normal fluid intake. (Measure your fluid intake, too). For each pound of weight you lose during the exercise period, your fluid shortfall is about 16 ounces. For example, if you lose 3 pounds during a two-hour training run, you have sweated away 48 ounces (3 lb × 16 oz = 48 oz) more fluid than you have consumed.

Your body can adapt to increased fluid intake, so during future training sessions, gradually increase your fluid intake—even when you don't feel thirsty—until you can replace at least 80 percent of your sweat losses during the exercise. In the example above, this means that you would need to increase your drinking during exercise by 38.4 ounces (0.80 × 48 oz = 38.4 oz). It's even better if you can replace your entire fluid shortfall, but don't drink so much fluid that you gain weight during the exercise. See Chapter 7 for more details on calculating fluid losses.

CARBOHYDRATE AND PROTEIN REPLACEMENT DURING EXERCISE

The primary fuel sources for moderate- to high-intensity exercise are glycogen stored in the muscles and liver and glucose carried to working muscles through the blood. Both glycogen and glucose are products of carbohydrate breakdown, and for this reason, they are often referred to collectively as "carbohydrate fuel."

Not all muscle fibers metabolize carbohydrate fuel in the same way. Type I, or slow-twitch, muscle fibers have a higher blood-flow capacity, a higher capillary density, and a greater number of mitochondria, making them better able to oxidize carbohydrate fuel (that is, metabolize carbohydrate fuel in the presence of oxygen) and therefore more fatigue-resistant. Type II, or fast-twitch, muscle fibers are better suited to producing energy in the absence of oxygen, allowing them to produce energy much more rapidly and making them better able to support efforts of maximum or near-maximum intensity. But these muscle fibers deplete their glycogen stores, and thus they fatigue, very quickly. During endurance-type exercise, use of type I muscle fibers predominates.

During sprinting- and strength-type exercise, type II fibers are also recruited. In both cases, depletion of muscle glycogen stores causes fatigue. A typical athlete's muscles can store about 1,500 to 2,000 calories of glycogen. At an exercise intensity of 80 percent of maximum aerobic capacity, available muscle glycogen will be depleted within roughly two to three hours. However, just a few maximum-intensity sprints lasting a few minutes each can result in depletion of glycogen supplies in type II fibers.

Blood glucose is available in much more limited amounts than muscle and liver glycogen, but it can be replenished much more rapidly. It takes many hours to replenish glycogen through carbohydrate consumption, while it takes only about twenty minutes for the sugars consumed in a sports drink to pass through the stomach and become broken down into glucose in the bloodstream. This is why consuming carbohydrate during exercise is essential for prolonging endurance. While an athlete cannot consume enough carbohydrate to completely halt the use of glycogen for energy, he or she can consume enough to slow its depletion significantly.

Studies have consistently shown that consuming the proper carbohydrate sources in the proper amounts can delay fatigue in endurance athletes and improve the performance of sprint and strength athletes. For example, in an English university study involving treadmill running to exhaustion at 70 percent of maximum aerobic capacity, athletes who consumed a sports drink containing carbohydrate lasted on average fifteen minutes longer than those who drank only water. Similarly, in a sprint-oriented study performed by researchers at the University of South Carolina, carbohydrate consumption prior to and during exercise allowed subjects to continue 45 percent longer during repeated one-minute cycling sprints separated by three-minute rest intervals.

The greatest performance benefits result when 60 to 80 grams of carbohydrate are consumed per hour of intense exercise. Research has shown that the gastrointestinal tract generally cannot absorb carbohydrate at a rate exceeding 1.2 grams per minute, and when greater amounts are consumed, gastrointestinal distress often occurs. Consuming less than 30 grams of carbohydrate per hour fails to take advantage of the muscle-glycogen sparing effect that results when blood glucose levels are maximized during exercise. Sports drinks that are formulated to take care of fluid, electrolyte, and carbohydrate needs should contain 6 to 8 percent carbohydrate to ensure that carbohydrate is delivered at the appropriate rate.

Physiologists believe that the muscles' ability to take up glucose from the blood far exceeds the ability of the gastrointestinal system to deliver carbohydrate to the blood. For this reason, once glucose enters the bloodstream, it is vital that it be delivered to the working muscles as quickly as possible. The hormone insulin plays a key role in this process. In response to the presence of glucose, insulin is released by the pancreas into the bloodstream, where it binds to glucose molecules and delivers them to the cells of contracting muscles.

Conventional sports drinks containing 6 to 8 percent (6 to 8 grams per 100 milliliters of fluid) carbohydrate produce a significant insulin response. Recently, however, some biochemists began searching for ways to reformulate sports drinks to stimulate greater insulin release, and they found one: protein. Like carbohydrate, protein is a potent stimulator of insulin release.

The hormone insulin plays an essential role in controlling muscle energy dynamics. As we have discussed, insulin is released by the pancreas in response to increasing levels of glucose in the blood and serves to deliver it to the muscles. Increasing the plasma glucose and insulin concentrations during prolonged variable intensity exercise has been shown to spare muscle glycogen and increase aerobic performance. Because of the critical role played by insulin in energy production, sports scientists have focused on how insulin might be stimulated during exercise.

As early as 1966, it was shown that protein could stimulate insulin secretion. In 1987, Gene Spiller and his colleagues from Shaklee Research Center, San Francisco, showed that a carbohydrate/protein mixture was more effective in stimulating insulin response than carbohydrate alone. In the study, fourteen healthy normal-weight males and females were fed meals containing a fixed amount of carbohydrate and varying amounts of protein. Average insulin levels produced by the carbohydrate/protein-containing meals were almost twice the level produced by the carbohydrate-only meal. Luc Van Loon and his colleagues from Maastricht University, the Netherlands, also examined the effect of protein on insulin. They observed that when protein was added to carbohydrate, it produced a synergistic effect on insulin levels. In a study by Ben Yaspelkis and colleagues from the University of Texas, it was found that during prolonged variable-intensity exercise, plasma insulin levels could be significantly elevated and muscle glycogen spared by providing carbohydrate supplementation. Moreover, K. M. Zawadzki and others from the University of Texas demonstrated that a carbohydrate/protein supplement was more effective in raising the plasma insulin level during a four-hour post-exercise recovery period than a comparable carbohydrate supplement. Consequently, this greater insulin level resulted in a significantly faster rate of muscle glycogen storage during the recovery period.

That these studies have strong implications for the exercising muscle is clear. Carbohydrate/protein supplementation, by stimulating insulin, should produce a faster delivery of glucose into the muscle, thereby sparing muscle glycogen stores and improving endurance. In a recent study by Dr. John Ivy at the University of Texas, ten trained cyclists were exercised on three separate occasions at intensities that varied between 45 and 75 percent of maximum aerobic capacity for three hours and then at 85 percent of maximum aerobic capacity until fatigued. On each occasion, each subject was given one of three supplements (200 milliliters every twenty minutes) consisting of water, an 8-percent carbohydrate solution, or an 8 percent carbohydrate/2 percent protein solution. Subjects receiving the carbohydrate/protein solution had a 24 percent improvement in endurance compared with those taking the carbohydrate solution and a 57 percent improvement in endurance compared with those taking water during the ride at 85 percent of maximum aerobic capacity until exhaustion. The investigators concluded that when protein is added to carbohydrate supplementation in a 1-to-4 ratio, there is a significant decrease in fatigue as measured by time to exhaustion. (See Figure 6.2 below.)

Lastly, a recently published study by Dr. Paolo Colombani of the Swiss Federal Institute of Technology reported that when marathon runners were supplemented with either a carbohydrate or carbohydrate/protein drink, the supplemented protein in the carbohydrate/protein treatment was absorbed and probably at least partially oxidized during the run without affecting muscle protein breakdown. Furthermore, no obvious negative physiological effects were observed as a consequence of the carbohydrate/protein drink during the run. It was concluded that the supplemented protein was absorbed and probably at least partially metabolized during the run and that no obvious negative metabolic effects occurred.

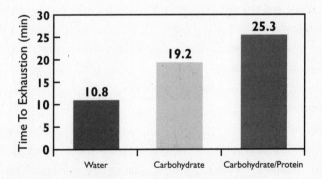

Figure 6.2. Time to exhaustion is increased significantly with a carbohydrate/protein drink.

What to Look Out for in a Sports Drink

The two main things to be on the lookout for when selecting a sports drink are the type of carbohydrate it contains and what "marketing ingredients" have been added to the drink to fool the consumer into thinking that the drink is loaded with key ingredients.

The types and overall concentration of carbohydrate have an effect on the physiological efficacy of a sports drink and on characteristics such as flavor balance, sweetness, and palatability, and these have an influence on the rate of water, carbohydrate, and electrolyte absorption. For example, beverages with too much carbohydrate often taste too sweet to drink during exercise, and therefore you won't consume enough to get the nutrients your body needs for maximum performance.

Commercially available carbohydrate sources for sports drinks typically include sucrose (from cane or sugar beet), glucose, fructose, corn syrup solids (often referred to as high fructose corn syrup), maltose, and maltodextrin (frequently, but erroneously, referred to as glucose polymers).

There are certain carbohydrate types, such as fructose, galactose, and polylactate, that if taken in large quantities have no positive physiological effect upon performance and can even cause gastrointestinal distress.

Let's take a closer look at some of the carbohydrates used in various sports drinks.

Maltodextrins

Maltodextrins are essentially a chain of molecules of the simple sugar glucose linked together. On average, about seven glucose molecules link together to form a maltodextrin molecule. The role

continued

of maltodextrins in sport drinks has received a lot of study—perhaps more study during the last several years than the role of any other type of carbohydrate. So we do know something about what maltodextrins do and do not do.

Some earlier research showed that drinks containing maltodextrins empty faster from the stomach than drinks containing the same percent of another type of carbohydrate, possibly due to a lower osmolality, which basically is a measure of the ability of a solution to draw water from other solutions. Osmolality is dependent in part on the number of glucose molecules and not their size. Because maltodextrins are a chain of glucose molecules, it is possible for a sports drink to have the same or even more energy or total number of glucose molecules and still have a lower osmolality. If the osmolality is too high in a sports drink, it may actually draw water from the intestinal walls. So instead of helping replace body water lost in sweat, it may actually take more water from the body.

Fructose

If a drink contains only fructose or fructose as its first ingredient, it could lead to problems during long-term exercise. The best type of carbohydrate for exercise is the kind that is easily broken down and absorbed by your intestines. The sugar found in fruit, called fructose, actually slows down water and energy absorption, hampering energy and fluid delivery to your muscles. Research shows that a drink made exclusively with fructose may actually upset your stomach. In addition, fructose has to be transported to the liver and converted to glucose before it can be used by your muscles or by your brain as energy.

A small amount of fructose in a sports drink won't cause problems as long as there are other, more easily absorbed sugars also

continued

present. Fructose should be the second or third carbohydrate listed. Most sports drinks will have one of the following carbohydrates listed first on the ingredient label: sucrose (table sugar), glucose (the sugar used by your body as fuel), maltodextrin, and some fructose. Simply check the label to be sure that fructose is not the first ingredient listed.

Galactose

Recently, a line of sports drinks has appeared on the market promoting the use of galactose as the secret carbohydrate to aid in athletic performance. Galactose is a sugar derived from lactose, which is found in milk. The manufacturer of the drink shows data in their advertising that when a galactose-based drink is compared with a glucose/sucrose drink during endurance exercise, blood-glucose levels stay elevated longer. No data presented in the advertisement show any improvement in performance or exercise time. Maintaining blood-glucose levels proves very little, especially if there is no data showing improvement in performance.

The data from a published study by Dr. Dorien Leijssen and others from the University of Limburg, Netherlands, shows that galactose is a slowly metabolized carbohydrate, and because it does not effectively contribute glucose to the muscles, it most likely leads to faster glycogen depletion—the complete opposite of what you want out of a sports drink.

Polylactate

Polylactate is a carbohydrate/amino-acid supplement purported to increase endurance. Polylactate contains molecules of lactate that are ionically bound to amino acids, principally those with more than two nitrogen groups, such as arginine, because of

continued

their ability to bind more than one lactate molecule. The first study on Polylactate examined its potential as a carbohydrate source and was conducted by Dr. Thomas Fahey and coworkers from Chico State University in California. He found that a 7 percent Polylactate solution was as effective at maintaining plasma-glucose levels as a 7 percent maltodextrin solution during three hours of cycling at 50 percent of the power elicited at maximum aerobic capacity. Again, as with galactose studies, there was no improvement in performance, only a maintenance of blood glucose. Also, there was no difference in perceived exertion, oxygen consumption, heart rate, or blood-lactate levels.

A more recent study by Dr. Thomas Swensen and others from the University of Tennessee investigated the addition of Polylactate to a glucose solution to see if it would extend exercise time relative to a pure glucose solution. In a double-blind and random crossover study, five subjects exercised twice to exhaustion at 70 percent of maximum aerobic capacity. During the trials, they consumed glucose or a Polylactate/glucose mixture at the rate of 0.3 grams of carbohydrate per kilogram of body weight in a 7 percent solution every twenty minutes until exhaustion. The Polylactate/glucose mixture contained 6.25 grams of glucose to 0.75 grams of Polylactate per 100 milliliters of water. The glucose drink was a straight 7 grams of glucose per 100 milliliters of water. At twenty-minute intervals, they measured maximum oxygen consumption, respiratory exchange ratio, heart rate, and perceived exertion. At thirty-minute intervals, they measured serum glucose, insulin, free fatty acids, and whole blood lactate. They found that the addition of Polylactate to a glucose solution had no measurable physiological or performance effects. In other words, it did not extend endurance performance.

continued

Marketing Ingredients

"Marketing ingredients" are ingredients that have a reputation for having performance-enhancing or healthful effects that may or may not have a bearing on performance. They are usually listed on the front label of sports drinks as a selling tactic. However, these ingredients are often included in amounts too small to have any physiological effect. Ribose, creatine, ginseng, CoQ_{10}, and L-carnitine are just some of the ingredients added to drinks in amounts too small to produce physiological effects. For example, ribose needs to be taken in excess of 5 grams to have any effect physiologically. There is a drink currently on the market that has less than 5 milligrams (1 milligram is one one-thousandth of a gram) per serving. The manufacturer lists the drink as containing ribose, which is technically correct, but it contains far less than the amount that can have a physiological or performance-enhancing effect.

Another sports drink on the shelves contains about 2 milligrams of CoQ_{10}, which has never been shown to improve athletic performance. It may have health benefits, but in that case it needs to be consumed in amounts ranging from 30 to 100 milligrams per day. When selecting a sports drink, make sure to read the ingredient label to ensure that the beverage contains physiological amounts of ingredients to improve performance.

PROTEIN AND BRANCHED CHAIN AMINO ACIDS (BCAAs) HELP REDUCE FATIGUE

Protein-containing sports drinks may offer two advantages in helping delay fatigue during exercise. The primary cause of fatigue has been shown to be depletion of muscle glycogen stores. By stimulating the hormone insulin, protein helps preserve muscle glycogen stores. In addition, protein may also affect other factors that play a role in the development of fatigue during endurance exercise, including the oxidation of the branched-chain amino acids (BCAAs). Whey protein is a particularly good source of BCAAs. It contains almost 23 percent of the BCAAs by weight.

Eric Newsholme and colleagues from Oxford University initially advanced the theory that fatigue during prolonged exercise may be partly related to exercise-induced alterations in the central nervous system. The theory suggests that as muscle glycogen levels decline during exercise, there is an increased oxidation of fat and the BCAAs leucine, isoleucine, and valine as fuel substrates. As a result, free fatty acid (FFA) levels in the blood gradually increase while the availability of BCAAs in the blood decreases.

The increase in FFA levels in the blood is accompanied by a release of the amino acid tryptophan from the protein albumin, serving to increase the level of free tryptophan in the blood. The result is that as one exercises, the ratio of free tryptophan to BCAAs steadily increases.

Increases in the ratio of free tryptophan to BCAAs have been shown to increase the entry of tryptophan into the brain. Increased concentrations of tryptophan in the brain have been reported to promote the formation of the neurotransmitter 5-hydroxytryptamine (serotonin). In animal and human studies, increased levels of serotonin in the brain and peripheral tissues have been reported to induce sleep, depress motor neuron excitability, influence autonomic and endocrine function, and suppress appetite. Consequently, an exercise-induced imbalance in the ratio of free tryptophan to BCAAs has been implicated as a possible cause of acute physiological and psychological fatigue (central fatigue).

One of the theories behind taking BCAA supplements (or protein high in BCAAs) during exercise claims that, by ingesting these amino acids, you can decrease the ratio of free tryptophan to BCAAs in the blood. As serotonin levels increase with exercise, perceptions of fatigue may increase. By ingesting BCAAs in protein sources during exercise, the ratio of free tryptophan to BCAAs is decreased; this is theorized to decrease perceptions of fatigue and perhaps improve mood. In general, the study results range from those that find no effect on exercise improvement to those that note some improvement. However, one thing is clear from these studies: Scientists must begin to compare various ratios of the BCAAs to see which combination may be best for performance.

There may be an additional performance benefit of BCAA supplementation or protein supplementation. During a study by Kevin Mittleman, seven men and six women performed two trials of rest in the heat followed by 40 percent of maximum aerobic capacity to exhaustion. The subjects consumed 5 milliliters per kilogram of body weight of either a placebo drink or a drink containing the BCAAs leucine, isoleucine, and valine. Those consuming the BCAA drink experienced a significant increase in their plasma BCAA levels. They were also able to exercise, on average, 153 minutes before exhaustion—16 minutes longer than those consuming the placebo drink.

When reviewing the data from these studies, it is obvious that the amount of BCAAs and protein given varies greatly between studies. However, since rather high doses appear safe, there may be a benefit in using protein in a sports drink to help reduce fatigue during prolonged exercise.

REFUELING WITH PROTEIN DURING EXERCISE HELPS MAINTAIN MUSCLE PROTEIN SYNTHESIS

The tremendous energy required by muscle contraction leaves less energy available for protein synthesis within the muscle. Furthermore, there is evidence that amino-acid metabolism and conversion of amino acids to glucose increase during exercise, resulting in a reduced availability of amino acids for protein synthesis. The amino acids utilized during exercise are derived from increased protein breakdown and decreased protein synthesis. The decrease in protein synthesis is related to the diversion of amino acids and energy away from the events supporting protein synthesis toward the events supporting muscle contraction. The increased diversion of energy and amino acids toward events of muscle contraction leads to the hypothesis that the reduced availability of muscle-building substrates may limit post-exercise muscle protein repair and synthesis.

The mechanical events of exercise also result in muscle structure and membrane protein damage, which translates into an increased need for repair and manufacture of protein. The availability of protein and amino acids is essential for this process to occur efficiently. Protein in a sports drink will provide an immediate source of essential amino acids, thereby possibly minimizing the degradation of muscle protein during exercise and maximizing post-exercise tissue repair and growth. It has been found that when a mixture of essential amino acids is provided before or immediately after exercise, protein synthesis is enhanced during recovery. Furthermore, when protein is combined with carbohydrate, plasma insulin levels are elevated, which reduces post-exercise protein degradation. Thus, a protein/carbohydrate drink may provide a substantial anabolic (muscle-building) stimulus during exercise recovery by virtue of its ability to promote muscle protein synthesis and slow muscle protein degradation.

GUIDELINES FOR OPTIMUM REFUELING DURING EXERCISE

In recent years, much has been learned about exercise physiology and metabolism. This new knowledge has led to many refinements in training and nutrition strategies. The newer sports drinks represent one category where the latest discoveries have been put to good use. Proper use of quality sports drinks gives today's athletes a tremendous advantage over yesterday's. Following are a few important guidelines for sports drink selection and use.

- The most important need during exercise is water. Through perspiration, one can lose more than 30 grams of water per minute. Due to physiological limitations, individuals cannot expect to replace more than about 80 percent of fluid losses during prolonged or intense exercise, but they should try to replace as much as they can.

This requires consuming 6 to 12 ounces of water or a sports drink every ten to fifteen minutes during exercise, depending on one's weight, the temperature, and the intensity of exercise.

- As little as a 2 percent decrease in body weight through water loss will cause performance to deteriorate; a 4 percent decrease can cause heat exhaustion. These facts show the need to stay well hydrated during exercise.

- In addition to water, electrolytes such as sodium and potassium are also lost in sweat. These losses also negatively impact performance. A quality sports drink is formulated to replace water and electrolytes in the same proportion they are lost in sweat, which is one reason sports drinks are preferable to water during exercise.

- Carbohydrate is the main source of muscle fuel during moderate-to high-intensity exercise. Depletion of this fuel supply is a primary cause of fatigue. Consuming carbohydrate during exercise has been proven to substantially increase endurance. Again, water contains no carbohydrate, but a good sports drink will contain carbohydrate in the amount of 6 to 8 percent (1.75 to 2 grams) per ounce. Some sports drinks contain substantially less than this amount and should therefore be avoided.

- The hormone insulin plays a crucial role in delivering carbohydrate fuel to the muscles. Research has shown that sports drinks containing protein in a certain proportion cause a greater insulin release and increase endurance more than sports drinks that contain no protein. The ideal ratio of carbohydrate to protein in a sports drink is 4 grams to 1 gram.

- Small amounts of protein added to a sports drink may reduce central fatigue.

FLUID REPLACEMENT

In addition to restoring your muscles' fuel stores, you need to ensure that you rehydrate yourself after exercise. For example, if you are 3 pounds lighter after exercise, you need to replace about 125 percent of what you lost, or 3.75 pounds of fluids, to ensure proper hydration. You want to overhydrate, because you will continue to sweat and produce urine during the rehydration process. A carbohydrate/electrolyte drink with protein is the best way to rehydrate your body.

Below is an example of how to monitor fluid losses during exercise for someone weighing 165 pounds who exercised hard for ninety minutes on a hot day. To monitor your fluid losses accurately, towel off any sweat from your skin and hair, and weigh yourself without clothing or in a minimal amount of dry clothing.

Weight before exercise:	165 pounds
Weight after exercise:	161 pounds
Weight loss during exercise:	4 pounds
Fluid consumed during exercise:	2.2 pounds (1 liter)
Solid food consumed during exercise:	4 ounces

The percentage of body weight lost during exercise equals 2.4 percent, figured this way: (165 lbs − 161 lbs)/165 lbs × 100 = 2.4 percent. Total sweat loss equals 6.6 pounds (4-pound weight loss during exercise plus 2.6 pounds of food and fluid consumed) or 4 percent of body weight.

In the above example, the person should consume about 132 ounces (8.25 pounds) of fluids over the next six to twelve hours to ensure adequate rehydration of the body fluids before the next day's workout. Remember, 16 ounces of fluid equals one pound.

Weighing yourself the next morning after voiding and being within one pound of the previous day's starting weight is also key to ensuring that you are not in a state of chronic dehydration. If you are down more than one pound, start sipping fluids before working out or competing.

CONCLUSION

The exercising muscle undergoes a number of fluid-level, energy, and nutritional changes that result in increased stress on the cardiovascular system, a decrease in muscle energy stores, and a depletion of critical nutritional components such as protein. Minimally consuming a sports drink containing carbohydrate and electrolytes can speed rehydration and help restore muscle energy levels. When protein is added to carbohydrate in a sports drink, it provides additional benefits that can help athletes perform at a higher level and recover faster. The bottom line—carbohydrate in a 4-to-1 ratio with protein should be an essential component of today's sports drink.

Replenish Glycogen After Exercise

In addition to restoring your body's fluid and electrolyte balance after exercise, you need to begin replenishing your muscle-glycogen stores. Because glycogen supplies energy in the form of glucose to keep your muscles working, restoring its quantities in the liver and muscles is an important factor in optimal recovery from exercise. How fast glycogen is manufactured and stored determines how quickly you will be ready to compete or train again at peak capacity. As you will see, stimulating insulin is the key to rapid and complete replenishment of depleted glycogen. In order to maximize glycogen stores after exercise, an athlete must also ensure that adequate hydration is also taking place in recovery.

INSULIN: THE MASTER RECOVERY HORMONE

Insulin is a hormone released by the pancreas in response to carbohydrate consumption. One of its main functions is to help transport glucose into liver and muscle tissues, where it is stored as glycogen. Insulin also stimulates the enzyme glycogen synthase, which aids in manufacturing glycogen from glucose.

As you learned in Chapter 4, timing is key in replenishing muscle glycogen. Your muscle cells are most sensitive to insulin during the first one hour following exercise. Assuming that enough carbohydrate is available, elevated levels of insulin in the blood after exercise speed up the transport of glucose to your muscle cells, and this accelerates the rate of glycogen manufacture. After two hours, muscle cells become more resistant to insulin, and remain so for several hours.

Clinical studies have proven that athletes who consume carbohydrate within one hour after exercise are more able to completely restore their muscles' glycogen levels. Athletes who waited more than one hour to consume carbohydrate restored about 50 percent less muscle glycogen than did athletes who consumed carbohydrate during the period of maximum insulin sensitivity. The most striking results were observed in soccer players who drank high-carbohydrate beverages between successive games. The players who had taken in carbohydrate were able to cover more yards in the next game, compared with players who did not supplement with carbohydrate. The lesson here is very clear: If you do not consume carbohydrate immediately after exercise, you will not be able to fully restore your muscles' glycogen stores—and depleted energy stores mean less energy for training or competition the next day.

During my work with the U.S. Cycling Team, as Coordinator of Sport Sciences, I tested this concept by having a group of cyclists consume carbohydrate immediately after the end of a training session. I found that in their next training session, performance improved and the cyclists did not feel as if they worked as hard. Clearly, replenishing muscle glycogen is of the utmost importance for optimal performance.

ENHANCING THE INSULIN RESPONSE

Because insulin is essential in replenishing muscle glycogen after exercise, researchers have focused on enhancing insulin release during recovery. Studies have shown that protein, when combined with carbohydrate, almost doubles the insulin response and increases the rate of glycogen synthesis by 30 percent. So it seems logical that any sports drink containing protein in addition to carbohydrate would offer an advantage in recovery.

However, more is less in this case. Protein stimulates a substance called *cholecystokinin* (CCK), which slows the rate of gastric emptying. Therefore, too much protein slows fluid and electrolyte replacement during recovery because fluids must first leave the stomach and enter the intestines in order to be absorbed into the bloodstream. Delayed gastric emptying slows fluid absorption and, as a result, rehydration.

The challenge, then, is how to gain the benefits of supplemental protein while avoiding the negative effect on gastric emptying. You can achieve this by carefully balancing carbohydrate and protein according to a critical ratio, which I call the *optimum recovery ratio*, or OR^2. When the ratio of carbohydrate to protein is 4 to 1, the protein does not seem to interfere with rehydration. For instance, if you consume 56 grams of carbohydrate after exercise, you would want to supplement this with 14 grams of protein, according to the ratio, in order to enhance the insulin response without affecting the rate of gastric emptying.

John Ivy, Ph.D., of the University of Texas, has conducted research on the effect of the amino acid *arginine* on post-exercise recovery. Arginine helps stimulate the pancreas to release insulin, and is also known to be important for muscle metabolism. Dr. Ivy studied the effects of carbohydrate supplements that contained arginine on the rate of muscle glycogen synthesis after exercise. Carbohydrate-arginine supplementation increased muscle-glycogen replenishment by 35 percent more than carbohydrate alone. Ivy concluded that arginine, when added to carbohydrate, makes more glucose available for glycogen production. It produces this effect by increasing the use of fat, rather than glucose, as an energy source after exercise. Simply put, arginine makes glycogen replenishment more efficient.

The results of these studies are meaningful for anyone who exercises. In order to rebuild glycogen stores, maximum insulin stimulation is essential right after exercise. The addition of arginine to carbohydrate along with the correct proportion of protein can improve performance by enhancing the insulin response, thereby promoting a faster recovery. This is illustrated in Figure 7.1 below.

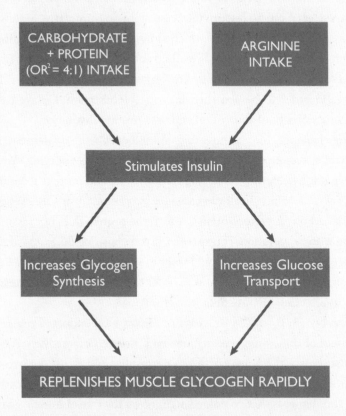

Figure 7.1. Stimulating insulin to rapidly replenish muscle glycogen

Assuming that you work out once a day for about two hours, you have approximately twenty-two "free" hours during which your body can replenish your muscle glycogen stores. Stimulating insulin without disturbing your body's other biological processes requires careful attention to your nutrient intake and balance. It must be noted that a high carbohydrate intake, above a threshold of 5 grams for every pound of body weight, will not accelerate the rate of glycogen manufactured following exercise. An ideal diet to replace glycogen and levels of essential nutrients involves moderate consumption of carbohydrate and protein. Fat intake should be minimized in the first two hours after exercise because fat, like protein, stimulates CCK, which has a negative effect on gastric emptying.

TAKING STEPS TO REPLENISH GLYCOGEN

Completely replenishing glycogen requires careful attention to your nutritional intake in the hours following exercise. Because your body responds to nutrients in different ways after exercise, it's important to balance carbohydrate, protein, and fat in the right proportions. And, as you will see, *when* you eat is just as important as *what* you eat.

The First One Hour After Exercise

It's important to note that the type of carbohydrate you consume plays a key role in stimulating insulin response. Some foods and drinks will cause a rapid rise in your blood-sugar level, allowing you to take better advantage of the increased period of insulin sensitivity during the first two hours after training or competition. You should select your post-exercise carbohydrate according to its glycemic index, which is an indicator of how quickly your blood sugar will rise after consumption. (See the inset "The Glycemic Index" on page 96.)

This is also the time to get a jump start on the rehydration process of bringing your body weight back up to normal from your sweat losses.

The Glycemic Index

The glycemic index is a measure of the effect of carbohydrate on blood-glucose levels. It compares the rise in blood sugar after a certain food is ingested with the rise in blood sugar after an equivalent amount of pure glucose—with a 100 percent glycemic index—is ingested. When you eat any food with a high glycemic index, you will experience a rapid rise in your blood sugar level, which causes your pancreas to secrete a greater amount of insulin. This is beneficial during recovery, because high-glycemic-index foods replenish glycogen more rapidly than low-glycemic-index foods. The table below categorizes some common foods according to their glycemic indexes when compared with pure glucose.

The glycemic index is important because it indicates the effects that different foods will have on blood-sugar levels. Many simple sugars, as well as breads and cereals, have high glycemic indexes. These foods replenish muscle glycogen stores rapidly because they cause an immediate rise in blood glucose, which stimulates insulin to speed glycogen synthesis and storage.

During and after workouts and competition, it's better to eat foods or drink beverages that cause a rapid rise in blood glucose, and an immediate insulin response, because they supply quick energy to working and recovering muscles. Other foods, such as fructose, dairy products, and some beans, have low glycemic indexes. You would probably not want to choose these foods immediately following exercise because your blood-sugar level will not rise as rapidly, making the conversion of glucose to glycogen less efficient.

continued

Glycemic Indexes of Common Foods

HIGH (GREATER THAN 85)	MEDIUM (60–85)	LOW (LESS THAN 60)
Bagels	Baked beans	Apples
Baked potatoes	Bananas	Applesauce
Bread, white and whole wheat	Bran cereals	Cherries
Corn syrup	Corn	Chickpeas
Cornflakes	Grape-Nuts	Dates
Crackers	Grapes	Figs
Glucose	Melba toast	Fructose
Honey	Oatmeal	Ice cream
Maple syrup	Orange juice	Kidney beans
Molasses	Pasta	Lentils
Raisins	Pineapple	Milk
Rice, white	Potato chips	Peaches
Rice Chex	Rye bread, whole grain	Peanuts
Soda (sweetened with sugar)	Sucrose (white sugar)	Plums
Sports drinks (sweetened	Watermelon	Tomato soup
with sugar)	Yams	Yogurt

If you're like most people, however, you may find that exercise suppresses your appetite. Even though you're now aware of the importance of consuming carbohydrate immediately after exercise, you may be unable to eat solid foods to replenish glycogen rapidly after a workout. Fortunately, if you find that your appetite is suppressed following activity, drinks containing carbohydrate and protein, in addition to their beneficial effects on rehydration,

continued

can help you to replenish your stores of glycogen in liver and muscle tissues.

Whether you choose solid foods or liquids, your post-exercise meal or snack should be consumed as soon as possible after training or competition in order to maximize glycogen synthesis. The optimum recovery ratio—about 1 gram of protein for every 4 grams of carbohydrate—seems to be the most effective in replenishing muscle glycogen. Try to consume 0.5 to 0.75 grams of carbohydrate for every pound of body weight, and include some protein in the proper 4-to-1 ratio. For a 150-pound athlete, this means supplementing with roughly 75 to 112 grams of carbohydrate and about 20 to 85 grams of protein during the first two hours of post-exercise recovery. Remember to minimize fat intake because of its negative effects on gastric emptying.

One to Four Hours After Exercise

You should consume another meal or a recovery sports drink with the optimum recovery ratio of carbohydrate to protein between one and four hours after exercise. Once again, whether the carbohydrate is in solid or liquid form does not seem to be important in terms of glycogen resynthesis. A high to moderate glycemic index carbohydrate meal will lead to a rather rapid increase in your blood-sugar level, usually within an hour. The meal should be composed of 60 to 65 percent of calories from carbohydrate, 20 to 25 percent from fat, and about 15 to 20 percent from protein. This will increase available glycogen for exercise the next day. After this meal, however, you'll want to consume mostly low- to moderate-glycemic index foods until your pre-exercise meal the following day.

Continue to rehydrate yourself. If eating solid foods, drink plenty of fluids with your meal.

The Remaining Eighteen Hours

During the remaining eighteen hours after exercise, and before your next workout, you should eat enough carbohydrate to equal a total intake of about 3 to 5 grams for every pound of your body weight. On light/easy exercise days, you should consume 3 grams per pound of body weight; on moderate duration or high-intensity days, 4 grams per pound of body weight; and on long endurance days or days of very high-intensity exercise, up to 5 grams per pound of body weight.

In other words, a 170-pound male would want to consume between 510 and 850 grams of carbohydrate during this period. A 125-pound female, on the other hand, should consume carbohydrate totaling between 375 to 625 grams. Again, the meals should include approximately 60 to 65 percent of calories from carbohydrate, 20 to 25 percent from fat, and about 15 to 20 percent from protein.

CONCLUSION

Whether you train or compete once or several times a day, muscle and liver glycogen stores must be rebuilt quickly. The speed with which your body synthesizes glycogen determines the amount that you will ultimately be able to store. And, simply put, the more glycogen that is stored in your liver and muscles, the more energy you will have during subsequent training sessions or events. Insulin increases the transport of glucose into your muscles and stimulates glycogen synthesis. This enables your body to increase its energy stores at an enhanced rate.

There is a narrow window of time during which the glycogen replenishment process is most efficient. You should balance your post-exercise carbohydrate and protein according to the optimum recovery ratio, or OR^2, which is 4 grams of carbohydrate for every 1 gram of protein. This enhances the insulin response without adversely affecting gastric emptying and rehydration.

Reduce Muscle and Immune-System Stress

"My muscles are so stiff and sore, I think I'll take today off." Sound familiar? Most likely. For many of us, these words are all too common. Sometimes it seems as though your body rewards your endeavors to stay in top shape with sore, stiff muscles in the days following a hard workout. And, to make matters worse, you may find that even though you expect to maintain good health by exercising regularly, you are more susceptible to colds and other illnesses. These signs are physical evidence of the tremendous amount of stress that your muscles have undergone, resulting in muscle damage and soreness, and even reduced immunity.

Although it is not possible to completely eliminate exercise-induced muscle damage, recent research has shown that the damage due to the stress of exercise can be minimized. This research has focused on the biochemical causes of muscle stress, and has identified several key factors that can help to neutralize a number of metabolic byproducts that are culprits of muscle soreness. In addition, various studies have pinpointed specific measures that can help you to enhance your immunity, which is often weakened by exercise stress.

FREE RADICALS AND OXIDATIVE STRESS

As you learned in Chapter 4, free radicals are highly unstable molecules that can damage muscle tissue. Because the rate of oxygen consumption influences the extent of free-radical damage, also known as oxidative stress, strenuous exercise increases free-radical generation. In other words, the harder you exercise and the more oxygen you take in, the greater the generation of free radicals—and the greater the potential for muscle damage. This is in part the cause of your post-exercise inflammation and soreness.

Free radicals damage muscle cell membranes by attacking structural lipids (fats) known as phospholipids. In combination with protein, phospholipids make up all of your body's cell membranes, as well as the membranes of structures inside the cells, such as mitochondria. The onslaught of free radicals weakens cell membranes and affects a number of membrane-bound enzymes. In addition, the reaction of free radicals with the membrane phospholipids releases toxic substances that can inactivate other enzymes.

Free-radical damage during exercise is not an issue to be taken lightly. Prolonged endurance exercise can result in elevated muscle and whole-body levels of free radicals and the products of their reactions. Fortunately, antioxidants are your body's powerful defense against these molecular bandits.

MINIMIZING OXIDATIVE STRESS WITH ANTIOXIDANTS

Antioxidants help to protect your body from the formation of free radicals. By neutralizing free radicals, antioxidants detoxify and protect your body against oxidative stress.

Your body produces some antioxidants as a matter of course. For example, *glutathione* is a protein produced by the liver from several amino acids. This potent antioxidant inhibits the formation of free radicals by neutralizing oxygen molecules before they can harm cells. And *superoxide dismutase* (SOD) is an enzyme that neutralizes the most common free radical, superoxide, and aids in the body's utilization of other antioxidants.

Your body does not produce some antioxidants, such as certain vitamins and minerals, so they have to be obtained from the diet. Unfortunately, even if you eat a balanced diet, it's often difficult to get from food enough of the antioxidants you need to counteract the effects of free radicals, particularly during periods of high stress or exercise. These circumstances may require you to supplement with extra antioxidants, such as vitamins A, C, and E, beta-carotene, and selenium. Two of these, vitamins C and E, are especially important for athletes.

Vitamin C

Recent research has shown that supplementing with vitamin C can help athletes reduce free-radical generation following exercise to prevent muscle and immune-system damage. It also aids in the production of anti-stress hormones, and is required for tissue growth and repair. Obviously, all of these benefits are of great importance to athletes.

One interesting study compared post-exercise muscle soreness in two groups of subjects. The experimental group was administered 3 grams of vitamin C each for three days, while none of the subjects in the control group supplemented. After the three days, both groups engaged in heavy calf exercise. The results of the study showed that subjects who had supplemented with vitamin C experienced less muscle soreness in the four days following exercise than subjects who did not take vitamin C.

In another study, subjects took either 1 gram per day of vitamin C or a placebo. Then, each subject completed a thirty-minute exercise session on the treadmill at 80 percent of maximum capacity. The test was repeated fourteen days later. On both the first day and the fourteenth day, there was a significant reduction in free-radical formation in the group taking vitamin C when compared with the group taking the placebo.

These studies make a powerful case for the importance of incorporating vitamin C supplementation into any training program. Many researchers now recommend anywhere from 250 to 2,500 milligrams per day to neutralize free radicals and to prevent or minimize cell and muscle damage. These amounts of vitamin C can be consumed in foods, in vitamin supplements, and in sports and recovery drinks.

Vitamin E

Vitamin E functions to improve circulation, relax leg cramps, and promote tissue repair—all of which are necessary for maximum athletic performance. As an antioxidant, it prevents damage to cell membranes by inhibiting the oxidation of phospholipids. This effectively prevents the cells' protective coatings from being damaged by the assault of free radicals. Vitamin E also enhances oxygen utilization by your body and protects other vitamins from destruction by oxygen. One study involving a treadmill test showed that supplementation with as little as 400 IU (international units) per day decreased muscle damage by more than 25 percent after exercise.

According to a recent report, vitamin E may be beneficial in preventing muscle soreness in people unaccustomed to vigorous exercise. William J. Evans, Ph.D., stated that vitamin E greatly improves the body's response to muscle injury. Evans found that 400 IU of supplemental vitamin E improved the healing process by increasing the mobilization of immune cells to damaged muscle cells, and reducing the production of oxygen free radicals. While Evans's study focused on older, active people, he concluded that younger, occasional exercisers could also benefit from antioxidant supplementation.

Researchers at Tufts University wanted to find out if vitamin E supplementation could reduce free-radical activity and thereby some postexercise soreness. As reported in the *Tufts University Health & Nutrition*

Letter, the researchers recruited physically active men between sixty-six and seventy-eight years old, and between twenty-three and thirty-five years old. Each day, for a three-month period, some men within each group were given 1,000 IU of vitamin E and some were given placebos. Before and after the supplement period, test subjects were asked to run 45 minutes in 15-minute intervals with 5-minute breaks.

The men were then asked to evaluate their soreness and undergo a battery of tests to measure biomarkers of muscle damage. What surprised researchers was that while the older men experienced less inflammation when taking vitamin E, the younger ones taking the vitamin also demonstrated less muscle damage and soreness.

Conclusive evidence of vitamin E's role as a muscle protector was also collected in a study performed at Penn State University in State College, Pennsylvania. In this instance, twelve weight-trained men were divided into two groups, with the experimental group receiving 1,200 IU of vitamin E each day, while the control group was administered a placebo pill. After two weeks, the test subjects completed a regimen of leg presses, rows, biceps curls, and squats.

The results showed that blood levels of creatine kinase (CK), an indicator of mechanical muscle damage, increased significantly in both groups in the twenty-four and forty-eight hours after exercise. At twenty-four hours, however, the increase of CK in the group receiving vitamin E was less than that experienced by the group receiving the placebo. This means that the degree of injury caused by strenuous exercise was markedly less in those men taking vitamin E.

Laboratory research has demonstrated that vitamin E can protect against loss of muscle mass as well. Researchers found that rats whose limbs were immobilized lost less muscle mass when they were given vitamin E as a supplement. This is akin to a person wearing an arm or leg cast and taking vitamin E to prevent excess loss of muscle. While a certain measure of loss is inevitable when muscle use is inhibited, vitamin E clearly prevents some of the potential damage.

So, what is the best dose for athletes of this powerful muscle protector? Based on the studies above, supplementation as high as 1,200 IU of vitamin E per day may be warranted to prevent muscle damage, although scientists have not yet determined the optimal intake.

Vitamins C and E—The Dynamic Duo

New evidence suggests that vitamin C works synergistically with vitamin E. This means that these vitamins have a greater impact when they work together than when they work separately. In addition to its multitude of other functions, vitamin C has been proven to protect antioxidants such as vitamin E. While vitamin E scavenges for dangerous free radicals in cell membranes, vitamin C attacks free radicals in the body. In this way, these vitamins reinforce and extend each other's antioxidant activity.

EXERCISE STRESS AND THE IMMUNE SYSTEM

Your immune system is responsible for identifying foreign and potentially harmful microorganisms that have entered your body and then neutralizing or destroying them. These invaders include viruses, bacteria, and fungi. White blood cells, produced by the immune system, are your body's first line of defense in the fight against intruders.

The stress of exercise affects your immune system by reducing the effectiveness of white blood cells and other immune cells. Exercise also depletes your body's supply of the important nutrients that function to keep your body healthy. The result is impaired healing ability and lowered defense against infection, both of which contribute to decreased ability to perform during training and competition. The situation is not hopeless, however. Evidence shows that supplementing with natural products can keep your immune system healthy. And exciting new studies have proven that, in addition to providing energy for exercise, carbohydrate drinks can help keep your immune system in top shape.

Glutamine: The Immune-System Builder

The amino acid glutamine functions as a source of energy for white blood cells and other immune cells. Low levels, therefore, may weaken the immune cells, which reduces resistance to infection. In addition, glutamine plays a vital role in helping to maintain the gastrointestinal system. Although glutamine is normally manufactured in the lungs and brain, both muscle and liver cells also have this capacity. This is important because your muscles store about 60 percent of this amino acid.

In times of stress, including the physical stress of exercise, glutamine concentration in your muscles and blood plasma decreases dramatically. This is partly because physical stress causes an increase in the production of white blood cells, and more of these immune cells require more energy. At the same time, the cells of the small intestine show increased demands. These requirements cause a corresponding decrease in your blood glutamine levels. Eventually, your body's demand exceeds its capacity to produce glutamine, and it must be obtained from the diet in order to ensure healthy functioning of the immune and gastrointestinal systems. Because the glutamine produced by your body must occasionally be supplemented with dietary protein, it is considered to be a conditionally essential amino acid. Be aware that although glutamine occurs naturally in a wide variety of foods, it is easily destroyed by cooking. Spinach and parsley, when eaten raw, are known to be good sources. Many sports drinks also contain supplemental glutamine in varying amounts.

Research with athletes has shown that endurance exercise significantly lowers blood levels of glutamine, which suggests that muscles cannot provide enough glutamine. Blood samples taken from athletes after high-intensity training sessions (between 90 and 120 percent of maximum capacity) revealed transient—but significant—decreases in blood glutamine concentrations. The same study also reported that after only five days of a ten-day period of hard training, glutamine concentrations were significantly reduced, even when the athletes were at rest.

Eric Newsholme, Ph.D., and his colleagues at Oxford University were the first to point out the correlation between strenuous exercise and amino-acid imbalances. A strict, strenuous training regimen that does not allow enough time for recovery may cause an athlete to suffer from over-training syndrome (OTS), which we discussed in Chapter 5. As you know, this syndrome is characterized by decreased performance, de-pressed mood, and increased incidence of infections. OTS has been diag-nosed in runners, cyclists, swimmers, skiers, and rowers, among others.

There is promising evidence, however, that glutamine supplementa-tion may lessen the effects of overtraining. Dr. Newsholme's report sug-gests that overtrained athletes may, in fact, suffer from chronically low plasma glutamine concentrations. This evidence is supported further by a recent placebo-controlled study, in which athletes took 5 grams of gluta-mine in the first two hours after a marathon. These athletes showed a 32 percent reduction in infection rate during the seven days following com-petition.

Most manufacturers of sports nutrition products are now aware of glutamine's benefits, and it has become fashionable to use it as a supple-ment in everything from protein powders to meal replacements. The un-fortunate problem is that glutamine is expensive, so many of these "enhanced" products actually contain minimal amounts. Some manufac-turers would like you to believe that a few hundred milligrams each day is adequate to maintain optimal concentrations of glutamine. In order to be effective, however, the suggested dosage falls between 8 and 20 grams daily, depending on your dietary intake, your health, and how frequently and intensely you exercise. Supplementation ranging from 2 to 6 grams, two to four times per day, should be enough to have a positive effect. One dose should be part of your recovery beverage. Larger doses will most likely create an excess of glutamine, which is excreted in the urine.

BCAAs and Protein Before and During Exercise

Strength athletes may not be the only ones to benefit from protein be-fore and during exercise. Triathletes, marathoners, and other endurance athletes often find that their own bodies turn on them, as immune func-tion is compromised and post-race illnesses strike. Reduced levels of circulating glutamine and other immune chemicals are partly to blame. To determine if this process could be prevented, Brazilian scientists led by Dr. Reinaldo Bassit gave male triathletes 6 grams of branched-chain amino acids (BCAAs)—60 percent leucine, 20 percent valine, and 20 percent isoleucine—twice a day for thirty days before an Olympic-style triathlon race. Subjects also took 3 grams of the BCAA mixture thirty minutes before the start of the race and continued to take 3 grams daily for one week after the race. Numerous parameters of immune response were monitored within the blood, including lymphocyte, cytokine, and glutamine levels.

A year later, each of the same triathletes received a placebo instead of the BCAA supplement, according to the same protocol. As reported in *Medicine & Science in Sports & Exercise*, results showed that when taking the supplements, the group retained plasma glutamine levels after the race; when taking the placebo, they were 8 percent lower. In addition, the supplemented athletes had fewer infections than the placebo group.

BCAAs are available alone or in high-quality carbohydrate/protein supplements or foods. However you decide to get them, they'll likely help you stay out of sick bay after your next triathlon or other strenuous endurance exercise.

Tips from the Experts on Staying Healthy

If you find that you suffer from frequent colds and other illnesses during training periods, don't despair! Scientists and nutritionists recommend the following measures to help boost immunity during and after exercise, and to reduce the incidence of colds and flu:

- Eat a balanced diet to ensure healthy levels of vitamins and minerals in your body. (For recommended vitamin and min-

continued

eral intakes, see Chapter 14.) Vitamin C in particular has been shown to reduce the impact of free radicals on immunity when taken for several days before long events or training sessions.

- Make sure that you get enough sleep, especially when you've engaged in several days of hard training. Lack of sleep has been linked to immune system suppression.
- Avoid overtraining. Remember that the key to peak performance is to train smarter, not harder. Pushing yourself beyond your limits can have a negative impact on your ability to exercise.
- Try to lower other stresses in your life. Mental and emotional stresses, including those from work and family matters, have been linked to suppressed immune function and increased risk of respiratory-tract infections.
- Avoid rapid weight loss during periods of hard training, because losing too much weight in too short a period of time can have a negative impact on your immune health.
- While training hard or tapering off exercise for an important event, it is prudent to limit your exposure to individuals who are ill. Research has also shown that heavy training is linked to suppression of neutrophils, the white blood cells that are part of your body's first line of defense against infections.

In addition to the guidelines above, you may want to consider getting a flu shot if you plan to train or compete during the winter months. Be sure to consult your physician to see if a shot is your best bet for staying flu-free during the winter months.

Carbohydrate: The Immune-System Crusader

It's safe to say that almost every athlete knows about the energy boost that carbohydrate can provide before and during exercise. But encouraging new studies have shown that carbohydrate can also help the body to combat the stress of hard training, which can suppress immune system function for several hours following a workout. Recent research by Dr. David Nieman and his colleagues from Appalachian State University in North Carolina has shown that athletes can lower immune stress by drinking a carbohydrate-containing sports drink. These results were achieved in subjects who consumed 8 ounces of the drink every fifteen minutes during exercise lasting several hours. Certain types of white blood cells associated with immune stress are increased in response to endurance exercise. Dr. Nieman found that this increase was reduced when the subjects drank a sports drink as opposed to an artificially flavored placebo drink with no active ingredients.

The same research team has also investigated the body's release of cortisol in response to the stress of exercise. Dr. Nieman's research found that cortisol levels were lower after exercise when the subjects consumed a sports drink containing carbohydrate during activity. Therefore, carbohydrate supplementation is believed to blunt the rise of cortisol in response to stress. Cortisol, as you remember, increases protein use during long-term exercise, which weakens muscles.

"Our research shows that sports drinks not only provide carbohydrate energy during exercise, but supports the link between sports drinks and less stress to the immune system," says Dr. Nieman. "Carbohydrate drinks of about 6 percent to 10 percent carbohydrate [per 100 milliliters of water] consumed during exercise will not eliminate the stress of training, but our research and the work of others show they can reduce the increase of several byproducts of stress and hard exercise." Therefore, carbohydrate can be a good addition to your antistress arsenal. Figure 8.1 on page 111 provides a brief summary of the principles of reducing muscle and immune-system stress.

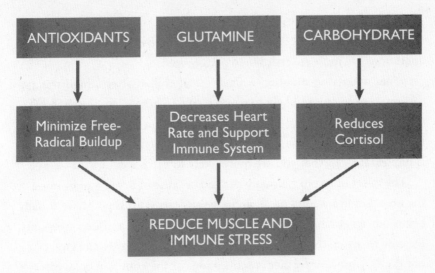

Figure 8.1. The key factors in reducing muscle and immune-system stress

EXERCISING WITH COLDS

Though it is relatively mild, the common cold is one of the most ubiquitous diseases known to humankind. It afflicts nearly everyone many times throughout their lives, some more than others. Even athletes are susceptible to colds, despite their occasional delusions that they are invincible to the frailties that befall nonathletes.

Viruses are the cause of the common cold. Incapable of living on their own, these small particles need the human body to survive. The virus invades the lining of the nose and throat. At some point, you may feel temporarily worse, with muscle aches and pains throughout your body as well as headaches. These more severe symptoms are usually caused by a brief run of the virus through the body. Rarely does your temperature stay elevated for a long period of time.

The primary factor that makes a person susceptible to colds, and something we usually have little control over, is exposure to a cold virus.

This can occur simply by hand contact with an infected person or contaminated surface. This is why individuals who live or work in crowded conditions are more susceptible to getting colds.

What about the situation when we feel chilled after a hard training session? Are we more likely to catch a cold? There is absolutely no evidence that cold weather, dampness, or changes in temperature will lead to colds. The only reason for not exercising on a cold, damp day is that it is unpleasant, not that you are more likely to catch a cold.

The onset of a cold is usually noticed because of dryness or burning of the nose. Later, a watery nasal discharge appears. At this point, we usually begin our treatment of nasal sprays, antihistamines, and decongestants. Despite relieving the symptoms, these drugs do nothing to the viral cause nor do they prevent further complications of the common cold. Most of the time, they make you feel tired and lethargic.

A cold should not curtail your training. If a cold strikes, increase your fluid intake, use a humidifier to increase available moisture, and take aspirin to relieve the aches and pains. Unless there are complications, you should be able to maintain your exercise program. Be sure, however, to exercise within the limits of your energy.

When symptoms progress to involve more body functions, special precautions are advised. If muscular pain increases, ear infections arise, and sore throat and colored nasal discharge appears, this signals that complications have arisen. Medical assistance is required and antibiotics may have to be used to fight the secondary bacterial infections. This is a time for rest and curtailment of training.

Fever associated with these bacterial infections is your body's defense mechanism of increasing metabolism so that your body will produce more antibodies to kill invading germs. Fever is the usual guide in telling you that your body is fighting bacterial infection, and you're better off resting, not exercising. Fever may be beneficial because many human germs grow best at the body's normal temperature of 98.6°F. Germs do not multiply at higher temperatures.

As soon as your temperature returns to normal, it is all right to resume your exercise program. However, you may be surprised to discover how quickly you lost your endurance. Studies on endurance athletes show that after ten days of not exercising, athletes lose about 10 percent of their endurance. The results may be more devastating after cold associated with fever. A study conducted in Sweden showed that colds associated with muscle aches and pains kept athletes from regaining their full capabilities for more than several weeks. It took this long for certain chemicals necessary for energy production to return to normal in the muscle.

Remember, as long as no fever is present, it appears safe to "exercise through" colds, taking care to exercise at a moderate intensity. Gentle exercise tends to break up the congestion quicker than complete rest. But keep the pace down to prevent coughing.

In the case of colds with fever or of the flu, more delicate care is required. A period of convalescence—first rest, then a gradual return to a full schedule—is a must. Don't exercise with a fever. After that, as a rule of thumb, take two easy days of training for each day of fever. Four days of fever and symptoms would need an additional eight days of recovery. Extended training that causes fatigue should be avoided at this time, or recurrence is a distinct possibility.

CONCLUSION

Many experts now recommend that you enhance your body's natural antioxidants, as well as your immune system, with vitamin, mineral, herb, and amino-acid supplements. Available research data has made it abundantly clear that these supplements are extremely important to protect your muscles and maintain overall health—and that most athletes are probably not getting enough. Given the evidence concerning the harmful effects of free radicals and immune-system suppression due to training, your best offense is a healthy, balanced diet, supplemented with a solid vitamin, mineral, and herbal defense. And don't underestimate the benefits of supplementing with a recovery drink containing carbohydrate, glutamine, and antioxidants after hard training to neutralize free radicals and give your immune system a boost.

Rebuild Muscle Protein

Through the years, protein has undoubtedly been one of the most widely discussed nutrients in the sports world. Some might say that it is also one of the most misunderstood nutrients. Bodybuilders believe that they can never get enough of it, endurance athletes generally don't get enough of it, and nutritionists will be the first to tell you that the average American diet contains far too much protein in proportion to other nutrients. In the face of so many conflicting viewpoints, how do you know if you're getting enough protein to improve your strength and performance—or even enough to maintain your overall health?

Fortunately, there are a few facts that we can all agree upon. As we discussed in Chapter 2, protein is a nutrient with various and diverse functions in the body. It is required for the growth, maintenance, and repair of all cells, and for the production of enzymes and hormones. And because protein is an essential component of muscle structure, sufficient amounts are required to maintain muscle integrity during exercise and for recovery after exercise to ensure proper repair and development of your muscle cells.

PROTEIN AS A FUEL SOURCE

The body tends to spare protein as a fuel source because of the nutrient's numerous structural and metabolic functions. However, when glycogen stores run low, some amino acids from muscle tissue are used for energy, even though the body can depend, in part, on the fat that it has stored. This generally occurs during intensive exercise, such as strength training or endurance activities lasting more than ninety minutes. Because protein is a component of muscle tissue, which is functional, this breakdown of muscle tissue has a negative impact on muscle strength and endurance.

As you learned in Chapter 4, your adrenal glands secrete the hormone cortisol in response to physical stress such as exercise. Cortisol extracts protein from muscle tissues in order to help mobilize energy for your body. As exercise duration increases, more protein is robbed from your muscles to meet your body's demand for energy, which, in turn, increases the need for protein consumption after exercise. By stimulating insulin with carbohydrate supplementation during exercise and recovery, the cortisol response to muscle stress is blunted.

BRANCHED-CHAIN AMINO ACIDS (BCAAs)

During hard exercise bouts, your body uses certain amino acids for fuel. The muscles use the branched-chain amino acids (BCAAs) isoleucine, leucine, and valine to supply a limited amount of energy during strenuous exercise.

Together, BCAAs make up a significant part of your body's muscle protein. In addition to providing some fuel for exercise, they are involved in energy production during exercise, and they promote the manufacture and growth of muscle tissue. Therefore, they are important components of the need for a carbohydrate/protein beverage during endurance exercise.

In essence, BCAAs are released from the liver and skeletal muscles. The carbon skeleton of these amino acids is used as fuel while the nitrogen residues form the amino acid alanine. Alanine is then shuttled to the liver, where it's converted to glucose (in a process called *gluconeogenesis*). Consequently, this glucose is shuttled back to skeletal muscle to be used as fuel. This mechanism by which blood glucose homeostasis is maintained is called the *glucose-alanine cycle*.

Thus, the ingestion of BCAAs may result in a net decrease in the amount of skeletal muscle protein that's broken down, which has applications to both endurance and strength athletes. Minimizing the rate of muscle-fiber breakdown is paramount for strength athletes such as bodybuilders. In addition, new evidence suggests that in a carbohydrate-depleted state, the ingestion of BCAAs may spare muscle-glycogen use.

Scientists at the Department of Biochemistry at Oxford University, England, examined the effects of sustained exhaustive cycling exercise on plasma levels of amino acids as well as muscle-glycogen concentration. Subjects performed cycling exercise at 70 percent of maximum oxygen uptake for sixty minutes followed by twenty minutes of maximal cycling (that is, the subjects were encouraged to cycle as hard as possible). Immediately before exercise and after every fifteen minutes of exercise, each subject drank a solution containing either 90 milligrams of BCAAs per kilogram of body weight or a flavored placebo. The two drinks had a similar taste.

The ingestion of the BCAAs resulted in a significant increase in blood and muscle concentrations of these amino acids, and muscle-glycogen concentration decreased much less in the BCAA group (about 10 percent) versus the placebo group (about 35 percent). Furthermore, BCAA ingestion resulted in a significantly greater increase in blood and muscle alanine levels. The researchers suggested that alanine might have been converted to glucose in the liver and then transported to the working muscle to be used as fuel. This would make sense, since less muscle glycogen was used in the BCAA supplemented group.

As we saw in Chapter 6, research by Dr. John Ivy and others has shown that the addition of small amounts of protein to a carbohydrate-based sports drink consumed during exercise can improve performance. Therefore, the ingestion of BCAAs and protein may diminish the loss of muscle glycogen and alleviate the loss of muscle volume, in addition to its positive effects on energy production.

DO YOU NEED MORE PROTEIN?

Many athletes are able to obtain adequate amounts of protein by eating a healthy, balanced diet. Athletes who engage in sports that depend more heavily on protein for energy, however, may need to increase their protein intake or use supplements to compensate for what they don't get from their diets. Some activities that require a greater quantity of protein for energy are discussed below.

Endurance Sports

Athletes who regularly push themselves to their absolute physical limits, such as distance runners, triathletes, and competitive cyclists, can seriously tax their carbohydrate fuel reserves. As these carbohydrate stores diminish, more and more protein is burned as an alternative fuel source. Up to 15 percent of an athlete's energy supply during prolonged exercise may, in fact, come from protein sources. In addition to this, protein is necessary to repair tissues damaged by the wear and tear of the exercise itself.

Heavy Physical Training

Athletes working hard in any sport for ninety minutes or more on a daily basis will also burn protein as fuel, causing them to experience the same wear-and-tear damage to muscle tissue as endurance athletes. Extra protein can help to offset tissue damage due to exercise and can provide a needed boost to rebuild muscle protein.

Heavy Weight Training

Athletes who engage in strenuous weightlifting need protein to repair muscle tissue that is catabolized during training. Extra protein also helps muscles to adapt to the progressive physical stress that is a natural element in training with weights. A weightlifter's body adapts to increasing stress by synthesizing more protein in each muscle cell in order to build stronger muscles that can handle more stress. A greater proportion of protein in muscle tissues translates into stronger muscle contractions. Therefore, the athlete will be able to lift the same weight with greater ease during subsequent workouts.

Sports Requiring Calorie-Restricted Diets

Wrestlers, dancers, jockeys, boxers, and others who have to deal with weigh-ins and weight classes often subject themselves to low-calorie diets for long periods of time. Unable to consume a healthy balance of nutrients, these athletes run short of glycogen stores in less time than athletes who consume sufficient nutrients to maintain their energy levels, and burn higher quantities of protein as fuel during training and performance. These athletes need more protein in their diets to replenish muscle protein that is burned as fuel, as well as to rebuild muscle tissue that is damaged during exercise.

Untrained Muscles

Muscles that are not used to a specific activity or level of intensity are more susceptible to damage. Therefore, athletes just beginning an exercise program, as well as athletes expanding significantly on their current program, are especially in need of extra protein. But be aware that any athlete who is trying to ensure adequate protein intake needs to eat just the right amount to minimize the formation of metabolic waste products. When too much protein is consumed, the body converts the excess to fat and increases the blood levels of ammonia and uric acid. Ammonia and uric acid are toxic metabolic waste products. The athlete's goal, therefore, is to maintain proper, balanced protein intake.

ENHANCING PROTEIN SYNTHESIS

The breakdown of protein for energy is a setback for athletes who have been training hard to make gains. When muscle-glycogen depletion causes the body to use amino acids as a source of energy, it cannot also use these amino acids for building and maintaining muscle mass and strength. The result is a slower rate of muscle development or even decreased performance capacity. In such cases, carbohydrate and protein supplementation may be just the formula to rebuild muscle protein. A summary of this principle is presented in Figure 9.1 below.

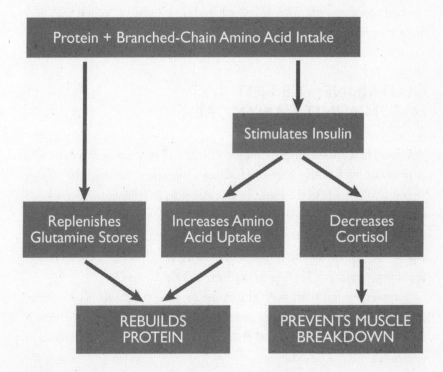

Figure 9.1. Rebuilding muscle tissues with protein and amino acid supplementation

The use of a carbohydrate/protein beverage (4-to-1 ratio) during exercise will also help enhance glucose uptake by the muscle, sparing glycogen, and will provide protein to help maintain muscle integrity and to use as a fuel source during extended long-term exercise.

INSULIN: THE JACK OF ALL TRADES

Insulin is an essential factor in maintaining a healthy protein balance. It increases protein synthesis by facilitating the transport of amino acids into muscle cells, where they can be used to synthesize proteins for structural purposes. Research has clearly demonstrated the advantages of taking a carbohydrate/protein supplement after exercise in order to increase protein synthesis. These supplements help your body to sustain an environment conducive to muscle growth and development, which carbohydrate supplementation alone cannot provide.

GLUTAMINE: IT'S NOT JUST FOR IMMUNITY ANYMORE

When we first discussed glutamine in Chapter 8, it was in terms of its role in maintaining healthy immune function. But since the majority of this amino acid is made in the muscles, it is also readily available when needed for the synthesis of skeletal muscle proteins. However, during times of stress, such as the physical stress of exercise, as much as one-third of the glutamine present in the muscles may be released to meet the needs of the immune system, leading to the loss of skeletal muscle.

Supplementing with pure glutamine or a protein high in glutamine during exercise is known to produce a strong anticatabolic effect, which counteracts some of the muscle breakdown that accompanies strenuous exercise.

High glutamine levels in muscle cells stimulate the entry of other amino acids into the cells. Thus, glutamine is considered to be an anabolic, or constructive, amino acid. In the scientific community, there is a growing interest in glutamine because of its activity in preserving muscle mass.

CONCLUSION

During strenuous or long-term exercise, protein—which is mainly a structural and functional nutrient in the body—is called upon to provide fuel for activity. This can have a detrimental effect for two reasons. First, amino acids that would otherwise be used to build and repair muscle tissue are instead used for energy production. Second, the physical stress of exercise stimulates the release of the body's stress hormone, cortisol, which breaks down structural protein so that it can be mobilized for energy. This results in a decrease in strength because some amount of muscle mass is lost. Recent research from several laboratories is now showing the need to supplement with protein/BCAAs during exercise to diminish the loss of muscle glycogen, to alleviate the loss of muscle volume, and to increase the positive effects on energy production.

Immediately following exercise, a rebuilding process is initiated to repair muscle proteins damaged during exercise. Recent evidence suggests that insulin is a strong stimulus for the muscle-rebuilding process because it increases amino acid transport into muscles. By blunting the rise of cortisol, insulin also minimizes protein breakdown from the muscles. In addition to this, glutamine is an anabolic amino acid that can counteract some of the muscle loss due to exercise.

Making Science Practical: The R⁴ Recovery System

B y now it should be quite clear to you that training isn't only about exercise. Recovery is just as important for performance. Why? Because the degree to which you restore your body's fluid balance, replenish energy, minimize muscle stress, and rebuild protein determines the level at which you'll perform the next day.

According to Dave Scott, six-time winner of the Ironman Triathlon, smart athletes take steps to optimize recovery by consuming the right nutrients at the right times, during and after exercise. If you guide your body's recovery with proper nutrition, he says, "you'll be a lot more consistent in your training, and you'll arrive at a higher level in your performance."

For years, many in the sports-nutrition beverage industry have looked at recovery beverages only as glycogen-resynthesis beverages. However, we now know through some innovative research that such a recovery beverage can be used as a rehydrator, a carbohydrate replenisher, a muscle rebuilder and protector, and an immune enhancer. In other words, a recovery beverage is much more than just a means to replenishing muscle-carbohydrate stores.

The R⁴ System represents an innovation in sports-nutrition beverages. What makes this model so revolutionary is that it goes beyond rehydration and carbohydrate loading to provide a comprehensive nutritional plan for recovery. The R⁴ System is based on significant studies conducted over the last decade, which have shown that:

- Insulin is the master recovery hormone that, when stimulated, can rapidly replenish muscle glycogen and rebuild muscle protein.
- Protein and specific amino acids, such as branched-chain amino acids and arginine, can maximally stimulate insulin when consumed in the correct ratio with carbohydrate.
- Antioxidants can minimize soreness and speed recovery by reducing free-radical damage, also known as oxidative stress.
- Amino acids and certain natural supplements can help reduce muscle and immune system stress during and after exercise.

By maximizing recovery with the principles detailed in the previous chapters, you'll find that it's possible to make great strides in reaching your performance goals.

Now that we have a better understanding of muscle recovery, the challenge is to formulate a practical program for the use of a recovery beverage that incorporates the principles of the R⁴ System for athletes of all levels and experience. The sports-nutrition market is glutted with products that guarantee to help you extend your endurance and increase your level of performance. But is the product you're using based on the revolutionary ideas above, or is it formulated according to twenty-year-old science? This chapter will open your eyes to what you should be looking for in a recovery sports drink.

THE RECOVERY SPORTS DRINK REVOLUTION

When it comes to recovery sports drinks, many manufacturers are only partly aware of what a product must contain in order to be truly effective. In the endurance market, carbohydrate and electrolytes have been much touted as the most essential ingredients in any sports drink. In the strength market, protein has been promoted as the Holy Grail of muscle recovery. The truth is that, although ingredients such as carbohydrate are certainly essential, numerous manufacturers have adopted the philosophy that more is better—which is not necessarily the case. For example, simply adding more carbohydrate without stimulating insulin may not be effective in rapidly replenishing glycogen stores, because insulin is a critical factor in transporting glucose to muscles for glycogen synthesis. And while protein is another fundamental component, some manufacturers include large amounts, exceeding the optimum recovery ratio. Others do not include any protein. As we saw in Chapter 7, some of these factors can have a negative impact on gastric emptying, which impedes hydration and electrolyte replenishment during and after exercise.

During exercise, you need a concentrated source of nutrient fuel that your body can digest rapidly in order to give you quick energy for that burst off the line or sprint to the ball. And you also need adequate fuel to keep you going for hours at a time. Carbohydrate and electrolytes alone are not enough to ensure adequate support of muscle metabolism during exercise to delay fatigue or to prevent oxidative stress. Protein is also needed in small amounts during exercise to diminish the loss of muscle glycogen and to alleviate the loss of muscle volume, not to mention its positive effects on energy production. And during recovery, you need a beverage that will enhance glycogen synthesis to replenish energy stores, provide protein to rebuild and repair muscles, and protect your immune system.

Several years ago, I participated in a conference with six leading exercise physiologists in which we brainstormed about what factors could lead to an improved and cutting-edge recovery sports drink. We reasoned that a product based on the latest science would offer major advantages over available sports-nutrition products because it would combine all of the benefits of the R^4 System in one convenient source. In addition to providing the benefits of rehydration and enhanced energy, the drink would be specially formulated to significantly improve performance by enhancing the insulin response to speed muscle-glycogen replenishment; by protecting muscle cells from free-radical damage, thereby reducing muscle soreness; and by rebuilding damaged muscle tissues with protein and amino-acid supplementation. The next step was to see how the R^4 System Drink would fare in laboratory tests. The formulation that was tested is shown in Figure 10.1 below.

	Restore Electrolytes	Replenish Glycogen	Reduce Muscle Stress	Rebuild Muscle Protein
Potassium	●			
Sodium	●			
Magnesium	●			
High Glycemic Carbohydrate		●		
Carbohydrate/ Protein (OR² = 4:1)		●		
Arginine		●		
Vitamin E			●	
Vitamin C			●	
Glutamine			●	●
Branched-Chain Amino Acids				●
Whey Protein				●

Figure 10.1. The R^4 System Drink Formula

WEIGHING THE EVIDENCE

Dr. Peter Raven, a professor of physiology at the University of North Texas State, along with Dr. John Ivy of the University of Texas at Austin, conducted the first study on the R^4 beverage concept. In this study, subjects were depleted of muscle glycogen through exercise and were then given either the R^4 System Drink or a leading sports drink during recovery. Following the recovery phase, subjects underwent a performance bout measuring how long they could exercise at 85 percent of maximum capacity.

The second trial was conducted by myself in collaboration with Dr. John Seifert, professor of physiology at St. Cloud State University. For this test, ten well-trained athletes completed a simulated duathlon. In the first phase, subjects ran on a treadmill at moderate intensity (75 percent of their maximum capacity) for forty-five minutes. The second phase was a ten-minute rest period, during which the subjects consumed either the R^4 System Drink or the leading sports drink. Then, in the third phase, the subjects cycled for thirty minutes at 75 percent of their maximum capacity. At the end of the cycling phase, all subjects underwent a time trial in which they completed a given amount of cycling work in as short a time as they could.

We found that the R^4 System Drink, when compared with the leading sports drink:

- Increased endurance performance significantly in subsequent exercise after ingesting a beverage based on the R^4 System versus a traditional sports drink. This is the most important aspect of the R^4 System. By the recovery process through rapid replenishment of glycogen stores, the R^4 System Drink significantly improved muscle performance. The subjects were not only able to exercise longer, but they also felt less fatigue, as evidenced by the fact that the ratings of perceived exertion were lower.
- Reduced the total buildup of free radicals in the body. The latest studies have shown that free-radical buildup is one of the causes of post-exercise muscle damage and soreness.

- Reduced muscle damage significantly greater than the straight carbohydrate beverage. As you will recall, creatine kinase (CK) is a marker of post-exercise muscle damage. CK levels in the R^4 group were almost 40 percent lower in the twenty-four hours after exercise when compared with the group that consumed the leading sports drink.
- Stimulated average insulin levels much higher than the traditional carbohydrate drink. Insulin stimulation is an important cornerstone of the R^4 System because of its importance in the post-recovery process. By stimulating insulin, the R^4 System Drink speeds the replenishment of glycogen stores. Based on recent studies, the drink appears to offer a benefit in blunting the rise in cortisol levels and repairing proteins damaged during exercise.
- Decreased average heart rate. By lowering heart rate, the R^4 System Drink decreases stress on the cardiovascular system.
- Produced equivalent rates of rehydration. Although protein, in combination with carbohydrate, has been proven to stimulate insulin, it can also slow gastric emptying. This is why the ratio of protein to carbohydrate is so important. The R^4 System Drink contains the optimum recovery ratio (OR^2) of 4 grams of carbohydrate to 1 gram of protein. This ratio provides the muscle cells with the benefits of protein without hindering the rehydration process.

Recently, Dr. John Ivy completed an additional study on a recovery beverage that contained carbohydrate and protein in a 4-to-1 ratio as well as the amino acid arginine. Eight trained cyclists performed two trials consisting of a two-hour glycogen depletion ride followed by ingestion of 12 ounces of a carbohydrate/protein drink or a carbohydrate-only drink immediately after exercise and again two hours later. Trials were randomized and separated by seven days. The 12-ounce serving of the carbohydrate/protein drink contained 53 grams of carbohydrate and 14 grams of protein, and the carbohydrate drink contained 20 grams of only carbohydrate. Blood samples were collected prior to exercise and throughout the four hours of the post-exercise recovery period. Muscle biopsies were taken immediately following and again four hours after exercise to determine muscle-glycogen content. Blood tests showed that ingestion of the carbohydrate/protein supplement resulted in a 17 percent greater plasma glucose response, a 92 percent greater insulin response, and a 128 percent greater storage of muscle glycogen compared with the carbohydrate-only drink.

New research, also coming out of the University of Texas, in a recent study published in *The Journal of Applied Physiology*, confirms the theory that the addition of small amounts of protein to a carbohydrate beverage is more effective for the rapid replenishment of muscle glycogen after exercise than a carbohydrate-only recovery drink of equal carbohydrate or caloric content. This is important new information, since some criticism of early research stated that carbohydrate/protein drinks used in the research had contained more calories per serving than the carbohydrate drinks and that may have led to the greater glycogen resynthesis after exercise. In other words, the criticism was based on the fact that the beverages did not contain equal calories. This new study shows that when drinks of equal calories are compared, a carbohydrate/protein drink is superior to a carbohydrate-only beverage in rebuilding muscle glycogen stores by more than 17 percent in early post-exercise recovery. Plus, you get the benefits of increased muscle synthesis, immune-system protection, and reduced muscle soreness from the protein in the beverage.

The lesson learned here is that protein (added in a 4-to-1 ratio) provides a double benefit. It enhances muscle-glycogen storage and provides the amino acids necessary to rebuild muscle protein damaged as a consequence of exercise.

FAST AND SLOW PROTEINS

Are all proteins the same? Are certain proteins better for recovery and muscle rebuilding? Dietary proteins vary in amino-acid content as well as in the amount of fat and other nutrients they contain. These differences can affect the digestion rate of a protein and the manner in which amino acids are released into the blood. Recent research has shown that ingesting the right type of protein following exercise may help stimulate protein synthesis to a greater degree.

Research has indicated that several factors affect protein synthesis after consuming a recovery drink or meal-replacement beverage, including the amount of calories consumed, the quantity and quality of protein ingested, the insulin response to the drink, and the digestibility of the beverage. The digestibility of a beverage is affected by the fat, starch, and fiber content of the drink, as well as the acidity. Generally, the higher the fat, starch, and fiber content, the slower a recovery drink or meal-replacement beverage is digested. The digestion rate influences the time course of amino-acid release into the blood. In this regard, beverages containing protein that are digested faster generally result in a greater release of amino acids in the blood over a shorter period of time. Conversely, drinks containing protein that are digested at a slower rate typically promote a smaller but more prolonged increase in amino acids. Different types of protein also have different time courses of amino-acid release. For example, since casein clumps when exposed to acid in the stomach, it's digested at a relatively slow rate, which results in a modest but prolonged increase in amino acids in the blood. On the other hand, whey protein is composed of a mixture of soluble proteins that are digested rather rapidly, resulting in a more pronounced but shorter increase in amino acids in the blood.

The time course of amino-acid release following ingestion of a protein has been shown to affect protein metabolism and synthesis in the muscles. For example, Y. Boirie and colleagues in France compared the effects of ingesting 30 grams of whey (fast protein) and 43 grams of casein (slow protein) on protein utilization and synthesis. The researchers found that whey protein ingestion promoted a greater increase in amino-acid levels in the blood and a greater rate of protein storage during the first two hours after consumption compared to casein. However, the rate of protein storage returned to baseline within three to four hours after consumption. Casein ingestion promoted a more modest but more prolonged increase in amino-acid concentrations that were greater than the whey group during three to six hours after consumption. This resulted in a greater amount of protein storage as well as in less protein breakdown.

The current thinking is that a recovery beverage should contain whey protein as its base to ensure greater increase of amino acids into the bloodstream, which ensures greater muscle resynthesis of protein. However, casein and other proteins should not be ignored in one's total daily protein intake. These proteins and additional whey protein can form a significant part of your daily protein intake.

Carbohydrate and Protein Post-Exercise Intake Increases Muscle Growth

Consuming a protein drink immediately after cycling dramatically stimulates muscle growth and repair, according to a new report from Dr. D. K. Levenhagen and colleagues at Vanderbilt University Medical Center. In the study, athletes were given a placebo drink (no protein, carbohydrate, or fat); a carbohydrate drink (8 grams of carbohydrate); or a drink containing 10 grams of protein, 8 grams of carbohydrate, and 3 grams of fat immediately following intensive leg-training exercise. Compared with the placebo, the carbohydrate drink did not alter whole-body protein synthesis during the recovery period; in contrast, the protein-plus-carbohydrate drink increased leg protein synthesis sixfold and whole-body protein synthesis by 15 percent. Also, glucose uptake by the leg muscles was significantly greater in the protein/carbohydrate group than in the carbohydrate or placebo group, showing a greater likelihood of glycogen resynthesis when carbohydrate is combined with protein. "These findings suggest that the availability of amino acids (protein) is more important than the availability of energy (carbohydrate) for post-exercise repair and synthesis of muscle proteins," conclude Dr. D. K. Levenhagen and colleagues.

SELECTING A RECOVERY SPORTS DRINK

When you select a recovery sports drink for optimal recovery, you should be certain that you get what you pay for. That's not so easy when you find yourself standing before a bounty of energy and recovery drinks, each one with its own remarkable claim. To help you narrow down your options, you can evaluate possible contenders according to the following criteria:

- Does the drink contain adequate amounts of antioxidants to be effective? Vitamins C and E, especially, have been research-proven to reduce oxidative stress and free-radical damage during and after exercise.
- Does the drink contain carbohydrate and protein in the optimal recovery ratio of 4 grams of carbohydrate to 1 gram of protein? Are these ingredients included in the proper amounts to maximize post-exercise insulin levels?
- Does the drink contain whey protein and the amino acid glutamine to help minimize immune-system stress and rapidly resynthesize muscle protein?
- Does the drink contain adequate levels of the electrolytes sodium, chloride, potassium, and magnesium? (Refer to Table 10.1 on page 132.)

An educated consumer is most likely to choose a product that suits his or her needs. Be certain to check the nutrition labels and ingredient lists for each product that you consider buying. This will help you to make sure that the product you select meets the criteria above for what constitutes an effective sports drink for optimal recovery.

CONCLUSION

The most up-to-date research has proven that sports drinks formulated to optimize recovery can help athletes increase muscle gains and improve

Table 10.1. Adequate Ranges of Electrolytes
per Twelve Ounces of Recovery Drink

ELECTROLYTE	AMOUNT
Sodium	75–250 mg
Chloride	45–75 mg
Potassium	200–330 mg
Magnesium	100–400 mg

performance. Few products are available, however, that can truly claim to maximize recovery. While many provide adequate ingredients for rehydration and nutrition for energy during exercise, they do not enhance recovery after exercise.

In order for any recovery drink to be effective, it has to stimulate insulin in order to rapidly replenish glycogen stores and rebuild muscle protein. In addition, a drink that is formulated according to recent studies will contain antioxidants to combat free-radical damage and, as a result, minimize muscle soreness. An ideal post-exercise drink, in short, should maximize recovery according to the principles of the R^4 System in order to minimize muscle fatigue, rebuild muscle tissue, and repair muscle damage.

Part III

Going the Extra Mile

Optimal muscle recovery is fundamental to achieving athletic success. By putting the principles of the R⁴ System into practice, you'll be able to replenish energy stores, minimize muscle soreness, and protect your immune system so that you can perform at peak capacity every time you exercise. However, there are measures that you can take above and beyond the guidelines presented by the R⁴ System that can be equally important in helping you to reach—or even exceed—your performance goals.

Part III will show you how to go the extra mile to ensure peak performance when you train or compete. It sets forth a complete guide to eating a healthy, balanced diet to maintain overall good health. This is followed by a look at the role of vitamins and minerals and then at some performance-enhancing supplements that can help your body to produce more energy and to build and repair muscles. You will also learn about effective methods of carbohydrate loading prior to competition to delay physical fatigue during your event.

The strength athlete has different recovery needs than the endurance athlete. Therefore, in this edition, we have added a chapter addressing the specific needs of the strength athlete. For years, the strength-training athlete thought that protein was the key fuel for strength and mass development. While protein is important, you will soon learn that the need for carbohydrate intake before, during, and after a weight-training session is just as important.

We'll also take a hard look at the nutritional and recovery needs of the masters athlete. As we get older, we need more of some nutrients and less of others, and the number of calories needed decreases slightly. Unfortunately, there has been little public knowledge on how the nutritional needs of older athletes differ from those of their younger counterparts.

We will also investigate the mounting evidence that athletes and active individuals need plenty of sleep. Fatigue tends to accumulate quickly if you don't sleep enough, leaving you listless, unenthusiastic, and susceptible to colds.

And, in the last chapter, you'll find an in-depth discussion on massage, stretching, and other nonnutritional methods for restoring your muscles to health and for maintaining muscle strength and flexibility.

Optimal Recovery for the Strength Athlete

The rate and extent of skeletal muscle growth that can be achieved by *resistance training* (also called *strength training* and *weight training*) depend upon exposing the muscle tissue to a favorable combination of training stimuli and recovery conditions. The optimum training stimulus for muscle growth is difficult to identify, although it certainly appears that high intramuscular force production is a necessary requirement. During recovery, the extent of muscle growth achieved is at least partly regulated by the hormonal and metabolic environment to which the muscle tissue is exposed.

There are two classifications of hormones that alter muscle growth—*anabolic* and *catabolic*. Anabolic refers to the process of building or synthesizing tissue, and catabolic refers to the process of degradation or breakdown of tissue. For example, when someone is said to be in an anabolic state, muscle growth is taking place. If someone is in a catabolic state, muscle is being broken down. The major anabolic hormones in the human body are growth hormone, testosterone, insulin-like growth factor 1 (IGF-1), and insulin. The major catabolic hormone is cortisol.

The following are the major functions of the critical muscle tissue–controlling hormones in the body:

- Growth hormone is responsible for bone, cartilage, and muscle growth.
- Testosterone interacts with the cell nuclei and increases protein synthesis.
- IGF-1 is responsible for inducing protein synthesis in bone, cartilage, and muscle.
- Insulin's primary function is to stimulate cells to absorb carbohydrates and amino acids, which produce energy and build protein.
- Cortisol stimulates the breakdown of stored energy such as carbohydrates, fat, and protein. Cortisol release is caused by stress (intense exercise, fear, or anxiety) or when carbohydrate levels in the blood are low and the body cells need energy.

BENEFITS OF POST-WORKOUT SUPPLEMENTATION

Recently, researchers examined the effects of beverages containing carbohydrate alone and/or carbohydrate and protein consumed immediately following resistance-training exercises. In previous chapters, we have seen evidence that consuming a carbohydrate/protein supplement immediately or up to one hour after exercise significantly restores muscle-glycogen levels.

The consumption of a carbohydrate or a carbohydrate/protein mixture following resistance training also stimulates an increase in blood-insulin levels. The increased insulin release is primarily stimulated by carbohydrate intake, but protein intake also shows a slight stimulatory effect. Insulin stimulates glucose and amino-acid transport into the muscle, as well as limiting protein breakdown. If insulin levels are raised immediately following a resistance-training session, the protein breakdown could be slowed, thereby magnifying the effects of protein synthesis and creating an environment for muscle growth. The effects of resistance training may be enhanced by post-workout carbohydrate/protein supplementation creating an increased anabolic environment.

Consuming a carbohydrate/protein drink after leg-training exercise dramatically stimulates muscle growth and repair, according to a recent report from researchers at Vanderbilt University Medical Center. In the study, a group of athletes were given a placebo drink (no protein, carbohydrate, or fat); a carbohydrate drink (8 grams of carbohydrate); or a drink containing 10 grams of protein, 8 grams of carbohydrate, and 3 grams of fat immediately following intensive leg-training exercise. Compared with the placebo, the carbohydrate drink did not alter whole-body protein synthesis during the recovery period; in contrast, the carbohydrate-plus-protein drink increased leg protein synthesis sixfold and whole-body protein synthesis by 15 percent. These findings suggest that the availability of amino acids (protein) along with carbohydrate are important for repair and synthesis of muscle proteins.

The presence of an increased level of amino acids in the bloodstream following consumption of a protein supplement and resistance exercise may contribute to an increase in protein synthesis. In fact, protein intake immediately after resistance training, instead of later, may be more essential for muscle growth.

Cortisol is released in high amounts during and after resistance exercise due to the increased level of stress put on the body and a decrease in blood-glucose concentration. If blood-glucose levels are maintained or quickly restored after a workout by consuming a carbohydrate beverage, cortisol release can be reduced. Not only does nutritional supplementation increase the amount of anabolic hormones released following a workout, it may also decrease the release of cortisol. These effects allow for an enhanced anabolic environment.

The optimal amount or type of nutrient to be consumed after a workout based on the existing knowledge should supply about a 4-to-1 ratio of carbohydrate to protein. Various drinks, mixes, and shakes available on the commercial market can be quickly consumed following a workout. A liquid supplement is absorbed quickly and allows the body to use nutrients at a more rapid rate. The key is for athletes to consume nutrients immediately following a workout to obtain improved results from training.

An athlete's nutritional intake plays a crucial role in the development of muscle size and strength in response to resistance training. A well-designed resistance-training post-workout beverage that provides both carbohydrate and protein has the following muscle-building benefits:

- Protein in the beverage increases insulin concentration and provides amino acids for protein synthesis.
- Carbohydrate quickly restores glycogen, increases insulin concentration, decreases cortisol concentration, and increases the muscle's absorption of testosterone and growth hormone.

In addition, a post-workout nutritional supplement can increase the number of calories consumed during the day. Providing the body with carbohydrate and protein when most needed allows for quicker energy storage restoration, increases the amount of anabolic hormone in the body, and decreases the amount of protein breakdown that occurs after resistance training.

Muscle Breakdown for Bigger Muscles

We often hear about muscle damage being normal with heavy resistance training. It is commonly thought that muscle needs to break down in order to promote strength and growth. A small amount of muscle breakdown is part of building bigger and stronger muscles. However, muscle injury to the point

continued

of serious soreness is not. New research supports the concept that resistance exercise disrupts, or "breaks down," muscle fibers. In response to physical stress, the body initiates a remodeling process to synthesize new contractile protein and make larger muscle fibers, and ultimately a stronger muscle. The small amount of muscle tissue breakdown following a workout is not as significant as when muscle is damaged or injured.

Steven Fleck, Ph.D., of Colorado College, and William Kraemer, Ph.D., of the University of Connecticut, refer to this process as "muscle tissue disruption" because the muscle can recover within twenty-four hours and isn't compromised in its ability to adapt to training. Workouts that cause real muscle damage lead to soreness or injury, as the muscle tissue is not able to quickly repair or recover. This is because the inflammatory processes are taken beyond normal repair requirements and can lead to continued cell damage.

Creatine kinase (CK) can act as a blood marker of muscle-cell disruption. The higher the concentration of this enzyme in the blood, the greater the number of muscle fibers with broken or disrupted cell membranes. When this happens, the muscle enzyme CK leaks into the blood. Muscle injury studies report numbers well over 1,000 units of CK soon after exercise and over 35,000 units twenty-four to seventy-two hours after heavy exercise.

Drs. Fleck and Kraemer have examined different heavy-resistance workout protocols from heavy strength training (five sets, five repetition max [RM], multiple exercises, long rest) to high-volume workouts (three sets, 10 RM, multiple exercises, short rest). Their research shows that most tissue disruption takes place with bodybuilding routines that create the greatest amount of muscle growth. Amazingly, CK values were only in a range of about 200 to 300 units twenty-four hours following the workouts.

continued

This clearly demonstrated that the amount of muscle tissue broken down in these rigorous workouts isn't causing significant muscle-tissue injury. The rigorous workouts were stimulating tissue remodeling or muscle growth. Even heavy powerlifting-type workouts only caused minimum amounts of cell disruption, with CK levels at about 100 to 200 units twenty-four hours after the workout.

Also, the CK levels peaked at twenty-four hours, which is different from injury/damage studies that have shown CK levels peaking anywhere from two to five days after stress. This means that the muscle is starting to recover within twenty-four hours. These new discoveries by Drs. Fleck and Kraemer make it clear that injury and damage are different from a good, hard workout. The remodeling of muscle is subtle and not a high-damage event, despite the associated difficult physical demands. They now feel that if a workout pushes one to the damage limits, soreness or injury may result. Their research makes one realize that if the workout produces a great deal of excessive soreness, the resultant damage may be too much for the body to recover from over twenty-four hours and may compromise adaptive ability to gain muscle size and strength.

DIETARY CONSIDERATIONS FOR STRENGTH ATHLETES

A balanced diet in conjunction with a resistance-training program aids the muscle-building process. Many individuals in resistance-training programs do not take in enough calories throughout the day to properly build muscle tissue. To increase size and strength, strength athletes must consume more calories than the body burns throughout the day. Excess calories are used for building muscle tissue.

In addition, family history plays a major role in the development of an athlete's physique. Athletes from families in which the members are generally thin are less likely to transform their bodies from thin, svelte figures to bulky, muscular ones. With improved nutrition and appropriate weight training, however, athletes can enhance that likelihood. Also keep in mind that as they age, many young athletes will naturally gain weight.

Body-Weight Composition

The primary goal of an athlete's muscle weight-gain program is to increase lean body weight. Weight measured on a scale indicates only total body weight and does not show how much is fat and how much is muscle. To tell the difference, it is also necessary to measure body-weight composition. One method to determine body-weight composition is underwater weighing. In this method, you are first weighed on a regular scale. Then, after exhaling the air in your lungs, you are submerged in a tank of water and your underwater weight is measured. The two measurements are plugged into a mathematical formula that estimates lean body mass and fat. Another method is skinfold measurement. Handheld calipers measure the thickness of fat under the skin on various points of the body. These measurements are plugged into yet another formula that estimates total body-fat percentage. These methods can be used to check muscle weight-gain progress.

NUTRITIONAL SUPPORT FOR MUSCLE WEIGHT GAIN

No nutrient or nutrient combinations from foods or supplements alone can induce muscle development. Increasing muscle mass is the result of an appropriate exercise program supported by adequate intake of essential nutrients, including carbohydrate, protein, fluids, vitamins, and minerals. The most important impact on muscle growth is taking in adequate calories along with training to ensure muscle growth.

Calorie Needs

The amount of potential energy in a pound of muscle tissue is approximately 2,500 calories. Linda Houtkooper, Ph.D., a nutritionist from the University of Arizona, estimates, therefore, that an increase of 2,500 to 3,000 calories per week (about 350 to 400 extra calories per day) over the calories needed to maintain body weight would theoretically provide the energy needed for a one-pound muscle gain per week. "Theoretically" must be emphasized, however, since there is marked individual variation in gaining muscle weight. The variation is the result of many factors, including the efficiency of calorie utilization, body size, body composition, and the type, frequency, duration, and intensity of the workout program. A strict exercise regimen must also be followed to avoid turning these extra calories into fat.

How rapidly can an athlete put on muscle? The answer varies from individual to individual. Since calorie needs and the rate of muscle weight gain will differ considerably, recommendations should be made on an individual need based on frequent monitoring of diet, body composition, and workout program.

The additional calories required for muscle weight gain should come mainly from an increase in high-nutrient foods (foods that contain vitamins, minerals, and protein as well as calories). High-nutrient foods include whole-wheat breads, cereals, pasta, low-fat milk products, low-fat meat, poultry, fish, vegetables, fruits, and recovery drinks. A low-nutrient food is one that supplies mainly calories from fat or sugars and contains very little vitamins, minerals, or protein. Low-nutrient foods include soft drinks, sweets, and alcohol. A muscle weight-gain diet should include calories from each energy nutrient in the approximate proportions shown in Table 11.1 below.

Table 11.1. Energy Nutrient Percent of Total Calories

Protein	15 to 20 percent
Fat	20 to 25 percent
Carbohydrate	55 to 60 percent

Carbohydrate and Fat Needs

Adequate glycogen stores (stored carbohydrate in the muscle) provide essential fuel for muscles undergoing intensive weight training. Regular intense strength training depletes limited glycogen stores. Glycogen is replaced mainly from carbohydrates in the diet. A high-carbohydrate diet will increase the rate of glycogen replacement and give you the energy to work hard in the weight room.

A modest amount of fat of 25 percent of calories to a maximum of 30 percent of calories (preferably from vegetable fat) may also be needed if energy requirements are greater than 3,500 calories a day. This increased amount of dietary fat will allow the athlete to meet energy needs without having to consume enormous quantities of food. Excess calories consumed as carbohydrate and fat, as well as protein, that are not needed for immediate use or for fueling muscle weight gain will primarily be converted to triglycerides and stored as fat in adipose tissue.

Protein Needs

Compared with carbohydrate and fat, protein is a minor energy source during exercise—it is estimated that amino acids in protein provide only 5 to 15 percent of the fuel for exercise. However, dietary protein's major role is to provide amino acids to build proteins, including those in muscle.

After conducting a comprehensive review of protein and its role in athletic performance, many scientists, athletes, and coaches have concluded that the RDA for protein (0.8 grams per kilogram of body weight, or 0.4 grams per pound of body weight per day) may be inadequate for individuals in training, in general.

During the early stages of training or during increases in training levels, additional increased protein intake may be needed to support increases in muscle mass, myoglobin (a protein that pulls oxygen into the muscle cell), and enzyme-content formation. Enzymes are important catalysts that speed up energy production in the muscles. The recommended intake of protein during this period may be as low as 1.2 grams per kilogram (or 0.6 grams per pound) of body weight per day. For weightlifters or athletes in intense strength training, recommended intake may be as high as 2 grams per kilogram (or 1 gram per pound) of body weight per day. In *Strength and Conditioning Journal,* Drs. Ralph Rozenek and Michael Stone, who have conducted extensive research in the area of strength conditioning, reported that a study of protein metabolism related to athletes indicates that protein requirements during strength training may be as high as 2.6 grams per kilogram (or 1.3 grams per pound) of body weight per day. Increasing food intake to meet increased energy needs will usually result in an increased protein intake that will meet the athlete's higher protein requirements.

Supplement Needs

In addition to increasing energy intake and maintaining adequate protein balance, supplementation with certain key anabolic (muscle-building) agents may help maintain or increase muscle mass. The advent of high-quality, well-researched supplements has been a boon to athletes, who had very few options just a decade ago. The following are just a few supplements primarily for the strength athlete that have received attention in the last few years.

GLUTAMINE

There is a growing interest in the amino acid glutamine in the scientific community. Numerous studies have shown its ability to increase nitrogen retention and preserve skeletal muscle mass. High glutamine levels in muscle cells stimulate the entry of other amino acids into the cells. Thus, glutamine is anti-catabolic and can be considered to be an anabolic amino acid.

HMB

There is no supplement on the market that has attracted more publicity in the last year than HMB (B-hydroxy B-methylbutyrate), which is found in muscle cells and helps prevent the breakdown of muscle. Recently, some human research has been done with supplemental HMB, and the results look promising. Several studies using both trained and untrained subjects on a three-day-per-week workout schedule who were given HMB found increases in muscle and decreases in fat. (More details on HMB are presented in Chapter 15.)

CREATINE

Last but not least, creatine, which is found in all muscle cells, has become a widely used muscle-building supplement since its use by many athletes in the 1992 Olympics. Creatine doesn't seem to have any negative side effects, unless you consider weight gain detrimental. Creatine is stored mainly in skeletal muscle as free creatine or is bound to a phosphate molecule (phosphocreatine). Phosphocreatine serves as an immediate source of energy for muscle contraction. (More details on creatine are presented in Chapter 15.)

MAXIMIZING RESISTANCE TRAINING

After strength training, the body is primed for nutrient uptake into the muscle cells. So, what should you feed your hungry muscles? Post-workout nutrition should follow two simple, practical principles discussed below.

Replenish Glycogen Stores Rapidly

Early studies primarily focused on replenishment of glycogen stores by consumption of a carbohydrate supplement both during and after exercise. Carbohydrate supplementation stimulates insulin. Insulin has two major roles: It facilitates the transport of glucose into the muscle cell, and it stimulates enzymes responsible for the synthesis of glycogen from glucose.

Recent studies have extended our understanding of how glycogen is replenished. A post-exercise carbohydrate supplement composed of high glycemic index carbohydrates (such as simple sugar) is more rapidly transported into the muscle cell in the critical post-workout period. (See the inset "The Glycemic Index" on page 96.) Enzymes responsible for the manufacturing of muscle glycogen are maximally stimulated within two hours after exercise. Therefore, it's essential that a carbohydrate supplement be taken within this time frame.

Even more significant are research findings showing that protein and the amino acids, when combined with a carbohydrate supplement, can strongly stimulate insulin levels in a synergistic fashion. As explained, the ratio of carbohydrate to protein is extremely important to obtaining this synergy. The optimal ratio should be about 4 grams of carbohydrate to 1 gram of protein. At this ratio, a drink delivers the benefits of carbohydrate and protein without negatively impacting the critical rehydration process. By further stimulating insulin with protein and amino acids, muscle glycogen is restored quicker.

Ensure Adequate Protein Intake

Evidence suggests that insulin is a strong stimulus of protein intake; it increases amino acid transport into the muscle and prevents the breakdown of protein. This interrelationship between glycogen replenishment and insulin is a cornerstone of post-workout supplementation. A second aspect of this process is the need for protein, glutamine, and branched-chain amino acids (BCAAs). Protein not only stimulates the replenishment of glycogen stores by activating insulin but also provides the essential building blocks for muscle.

Finally, carbohydrate with protein is the key nutrient combination for muscle growth. Supplements containing primarily protein are not the best choice for a recovery beverage after a hard session of resistance training. Carbohydrate with moderate protein and glutamine is the best recovery beverage for muscle recovery and growth—whether you are an endurance athlete or a strength athlete.

CARBOHYDRATE AND PROTEIN BEFORE AND DURING STRENGTH-TRAINING WORKOUTS

Conventional gym wisdom in the past has been that carbohydrate/protein and protein supplements should be taken immediately after a weight-training workout. As we discussed earlier, the idea behind taking a carbohydrate/protein supplement after a workout is that the workout creates a stimulus for muscle carbohydrate and protein synthesis, which results in rebuilding energy stores and gains in muscle mass. So, by taking a carbohydrate/protein supplement right after a workout, the carbohydrate and amino acids necessary for protein synthesis are available for muscle repair and the building of new muscle mass.

Carbohydrate is also critical for muscle contraction and delaying muscle fatigue, especially during stressful exercise. Protein and essential amino acid availability is vital *before* a workout, as well. This can help decrease muscle breakdown and has a positive effect on muscle building. Creating an anabolic environment for muscle growth (increasing protein synthesis while lowering protein breakdown) sounds simple enough. What's interesting is that one of the signals for stimulating protein synthesis is availability of essential amino acids and their concentrations outside the cells.

In one recent study published in the Canadian *Journal of Applied Physiology*, Dr. Robert Wolfe shows that drinking a carbohydrate/protein beverage *before and during* a weight-training workout is as effective at increasing protein synthesis as drinking a carbohydrate/protein beverage *after* a workout. The reasons are not entirely clear but may be related to the amino acids creating an anabolic, or muscle-building, stimulus. Then, when the stimulus of the training session occurs, there's a synergistic effect resulting in greater protein synthesis. Greater muscle protein synthesis over time will result in greater muscle mass. Although more research is needed concerning the timing of protein supplements, taking a carbohydrate/protein supplement in a 4-to-1 ratio prior to and during a workout may be as advantageous as supplementing after a workout.

The superior anabolic effect observed when a carbohydrate/protein drink is consumed before exercise probably reflects a greater delivery of amino acids to the muscle, due to the increase in blood flow that occurs during exercise. This apparently enables more amino acids to be taken up by the muscles and seems to promote greater muscle-protein synthesis.

Bottom line? The alliance of protein and carbohydrates with resistance training creates a substantial anabolic effect.

CONCLUSION

For quite some time, the strength-training athlete had believed that protein was the key fuel for strength and mass development. However, while protein is important, the need for carbohydrate intake before, during, and after weight-training is just as important.

In strength sports, carbohydrate (glycogen) provides the fuel to allow one to lift the weights in the gym. Without an adequate amount of carbohydrate, there is not enough energy to perform well or to maximum capacity. This negatively affects strength development.

Strength athletes must realize that once they reach about 1 to 1.3 grams of protein intake per pound of body weight on a daily basis, they are taking in too much protein, and that this has no physiological impact on building strength and muscle mass. The proper ratio of carbohydrate to protein (4 to 1) leads to greater strength gains in the long run.

Recovery for the Masters Athlete

Forty? Fifty? Sixty? Did you ever think you would reach those years? You and your training partners are on the leading edge of a change in this country—a movement of increasing participation in sports by people forty years of age and older. Continued participation in sports is increasingly popular because our society's attitude about aging is changing. The new crop of forty-, fifty-, and sixty-year-olds are far more likely to stay involved in their sports than were their predecessors. Society's interest in health, fitness, nutrition, and athletics is at an all-time high, and that support buoys participation by all ages. Media coverage of masters and seniors competitions is increasing, and athletes who gained recognition in their younger years are still catching headlines as they compete in their later years. The increased number of age-group competitions in many sports also keeps masters athletes training and competing.

Whatever your reason, training and competing have become your passion. It's hard to imagine life without a good workout and an occasional race. Being fit is both emotionally and physically rewarding. It is also challenging.

Most of us would agree that lifelong good health is one of our long-term goals. Neglecting to take care of ourselves is penny-wise and pound-foolish. Exercise, good nutrition, and proper supplementation have plenty of immediate benefits as well. Physically fit people tend to have more energy. They feel more relaxed, so they can think more clearly and manage stress better. Exercise, a good diet, and the use of supplements helps them to look and feel good.

A well-balanced training program, eating right, and the correct use of supplements are all necessary to be successful in your athletic endeavors.

MUSCLE MASS AND PHYSICAL CAPACITY

Muscles function as the engines of the body, releasing energy, producing power, and performing movement. Consequently, loss of muscle reduces the capacity to work, play, and carry on everyday activities. In a sense, the aging process is analogous to the power loss you would experience moving from a vehicle with an eight-cylinder engine to one with a six-cylinder engine and then to one with a four-cylinder engine. It's like starting out with a finely tuned race car and ending up with a worn-out used car.

Fortunately, the ability to increase muscle mass and physical capacity is not limited to young adults. In one study, men between sixty and seventy-two years of age were examined before and after twelve weeks of strength training. The thirty-six exercise sessions produced in participants a 9 percent increase in quadricep muscle size, and more than a 100 percent increase in leg strength. Although it is not possible for a seventy-year-old to function as well as he did when he was twenty, it is encouraging to know that muscle size and strength can be improved at any age through minimal strength training—in as little as twenty minutes, three times a week.

METABOLIC FUNCTION

In addition to enhancing physical appearance and physical capacity, muscle mass is closely related to our resting metabolic rate (the rate at which we burn calories). A half-pound per year loss of muscle tissue starting around age thirty is largely responsible for the gradual reduction in resting metabolism associated with the aging process. Research in the 1970s revealed a 3 to 5 percent decrease per decade in resting metabolic rate among nonexercising men after age thirty.

Muscle, a very active tissue, has high-energy requirements in order to provide for protein synthesis and rebuilding. And this ongoing maintenance effort is costly: every pound of muscle utilizes some fifty calories per day at rest. Because muscle loss and metabolic reduction go hand-in-hand, if you choose not to work out using resistance exercises, you should cut back at the dinner table. Just as a Volkswagen engine requires less gas than a Corvette engine, smaller muscles require fewer calories than do larger muscles. This is just as true during rest as during activity. Even when we're asleep, our skeletal muscles account for more than one-quarter of our total calorie utilization.

It appears that much of the slowing that occurs after age forty or fifty is due not to age, but rather to a lack of activity and poor nutrition. There is growing evidence that Jack LaLanne's saying "Use it or lose it" is firmly grounded in science. Most of that loss is due to inactivity, and some to poor nutrition and supplementation.

The answer is not to slow down. Aging need not be characterized by poor health and rapidly declining fitness. Vigor, good nutrition, and supplementation are strong medicines. Take them on a daily basis. By maintaining an active lifestyle, you will not only burn more calories on a daily basis but also maintain more muscle mass.

MINIMIZING INJURIES WITH RECOVERY TIME AND PROPER NUTRITION

Although some athletes pride themselves on not having missed a day in their training for the past ten or fifteen years, for most of us, training seven days a week is a sure route to early retirement from the sport. Many top masters athletes come and go, one year breaking records and winning medals, the next year so hobbled that they abandon competition or even stop training altogether.

One rule of physiology is true for the masters athlete: As we age, we need more recovery time. Recovery time can come in one of two forms: easy workouts following hard workouts, or rest days. We should schedule at least one full rest day into our weekly workout schedule; for some of us, two days of complete rest from physical activities are necessary.

Former Oregon track coach Bill Bowerman rightfully received credit for initiating the hard-easy approach to training: first day, train hard; second day, rest. But Bowerman didn't limit rest to one day, often prescribing two or three days of rest after particularly stressful workouts. Some older athletes will be able to get away with one full rest day plus one semi-rest day per week. The semi-rest day may involve some other aerobic activity or strength-training exercise.

Keep a journal to track the results of your hard workouts, easy workouts, and rest days. Pay attention to how quickly or how slowly you recover from a hard workout, and adjust your schedule accordingly. It is important to realize that even on a day in which you are training, your body is working to recover from its last hard workout. If you ignore the need for rest, injury will be your constant companion.

Overall, masters athletes need to moderate their training, take rest days, and use proper nutrition and supplementation to ensure adequate recovery and repair of muscles, tendons, ligaments, and joints. Injuries (both internal and external) can heal faster and better when the body gets all the nutrients it needs to rebuild and strengthen damaged connective tissue and help with the reduction of inflammation. To rebuild, we literally need "building blocks" to do the job. Nutritional research has pinpointed the very enzymes, minerals, amino acids, and vitamins that the body uses to heal. They are involved in the rebuilding of skin, tendons, ligaments, cartilage, and even the bone matrix.

MASTERS ATHLETES' DIETARY NEEDS

Most nutritionists agree that masters athletes should follow the same sound nutritional diet that is recommended for other active athletes, but they underline that advice by adding that as people get older, they sometimes fail to absorb vitamins and minerals from food as well as they did when they were younger. Therefore, it's even more important for masters athletes to choose high-quality foods than it is for young athletes.

Sometimes, younger athletes can get away with junk-food diets, but older athletes should be particularly careful as the nutrients they take in are less well absorbed the older they get. Choosing high-quality foods fits into a good-health approach. As we get older, we become more concerned about heart health and high blood pressure. A good sports diet is also a heart-healthy diet.

Some aging athletes take wholesome foods for granted and turn to dietary supplements, such as DHEA, androstenedione, and human growth hormone releasers, hoping to find that magic pill that will bring peak performance. There are many promising supplements on the market, some of which boost strength and endurance; however, none are as powerful as a nutrient-dense diet.

The bottom line on nutrition for the mature athlete is very simple: Pause a moment before eating anything and objectively analyze what the end result will be of the food you're about to put into your mouth. Will it enhance your training or contribute to good health? Will it help maintain muscle mass? Or will it leave behind empty calories looking for a thigh on which to take up residence?

Also, keep in mind that as we age, we do not need the volume of food we did twenty-five or thirty years ago. Your adolescent growth spurts, which required large amounts of calories, are long behind you. Yes, your training and competition requires a large expenditure of calories, but you still have to be very careful about monitoring the number of calories you consume on a daily basis.

MINIMIZING THE EFFECTS OF AGING WITH ENDURANCE TRAINING AND STRENGTH TRAINING

Because bone density and muscle mass are directly related, untrained muscles may be responsible for the number of musculoskeletal problems so common in older men and women. Consider the fact that four out of five adults experience lower back discomfort. When you also consider that about 80 percent of all low-back pain is muscular in nature, you get some idea of how valuable strength training can be. In an interesting study along these lines, 80 percent of low-back pain sufferers were symptom-free after several weeks of back-strengthening exercises. And other studies suggest, although substantiating research is still pending, that strength training may also benefit sufferers of osteoporosis and other degenerative diseases.

So where does all this leave us? The bad news is that research verifies what we already know. As we age, we typically experience a gradual decline in our cardiovascular endurance, muscular strength, muscle mass, physical capacity, and metabolic function. These changes increase our risk of cardiovascular disease, musculoskeletal injury, and various degenerative disorders. The good news is that regardless of age, with regular endurance exercise and sensible strength training, we can reverse these insidious processes and delay the debilitating effects of aging. The message is clear: Considering the relatively low investment in time and the high dividends in physical fitness, we should all be participating regularly in appropriate levels of endurance and strength training.

RELIEVING JOINT PAIN AND ARTHRITIS

Do your joints ache at the end of a run? Did you injure the cartilage in one or both of your knees during a previous incarnation as a soccer or softball player? Have you been told that you have a degenerative joint disease? Too much wear and tear can lead to osteoarthritis, sports injuries, and further loss of bone and joint function.

Painkillers like acetaminophen and nonsteroidal anti-inflammatory drugs, including aspirin, are commonly used to treat sports injuries and osteoarthritis, but pain relief and improved movement in chronically sore joints is only temporary. Chronic dosing is often necessary to obtain relief, and these painkillers can all cause serious adverse effects, such as ulceration of the stomach and duodenum, digestive-tract bleeding, toxic effects on the liver, and risk of kidney problems. Fortunately, certain nutritional strategies may keep your joints happier and healthier, helping you train pain-free for years to come.

How do you know if your joints need specific nutrients that they aren't already getting? There is no cut-and-dried test that detects a deficiency of nutrient X or Y in your knee joint. However, there is plenty of research that illustrates which nutrients directly impact joint health.

Each nutrient's role becomes clear if we look at what makes a joint function well or poorly. We know that healthy cartilage is a key to maintaining healthy joints. Let's take a look at some of the more popular supplements used to relieve joint pain and arthritis.

Glucosamine

Glucosamine is a simple molecule that the body makes from sugar and uses as a major building block of cartilage. It stimulates cartilage cells to synthesize the ingredients for more cartilage. In a handful of good studies in Europe, osteoarthritis sufferers who took 1,500 milligrams of glucosamine each day for one to three months reported less pain, swelling, and tenderness than those who took a placebo. Many experienced as much relief as those who took painkilling drugs.

In one study of 200 people with arthritis of the knees, glucosamine matched the popular painkiller ibuprofen, the active ingredient in Advil and Motrin. Each relieved symptoms in about half of the 100 people who took it. But after four weeks, those in the ibuprofen group were six times more likely than those in the glucosamine group to report side effects like heartburn, stomach pain, and nausea or to stop taking their medication.

If you are interested, I suggest that you try 500 milligrams of glucosamine three times a day for a month; if you notice a decrease in symptoms, you can continue for as long as it seems to work and there are no uncomfortable side effects. If there's no relief after four weeks—and studies report that this happens in 20 to 50 percent of people—you can stop taking glucosamine.

Chondroitin

Chondroitin sulfate is another one of the molecules that make up cartilage. One of its functions is to draw fluid into the tissue, which gives the cartilage resistance and elasticity. Like glucosamine, chondroitin stimulates cartilage cells to form the components of new cartilage, at least in test tubes. It may also slow the breakdown of cartilage.

In one of four published well-designed studies, Pietro Morreale and colleagues in Italy and Switzerland tested 1,200 milligrams of chondroitin sulfate a day for three months against either 150 milligrams of the popular prescription pain reliever diclofenac sodium (Voltaren) or a placebo. Among the 146 volunteers, who all had arthritis of the knees, those taking chondroitin reported as much pain relief as those taking the drug. Both groups experienced more relief than people who were given a placebo.

Chondroitin and Glucosamine

If glucosamine and chondroitin each make life more bearable for people with arthritis and sore joints, will glucosamine plus chondroitin lead to double relief? So far, just one study has tested the two supplements together, but it didn't compare their impact to either one alone. A study of thirty-four Navy SEALs and divers—who are at high risk for arthritis—received either a daily combination of 1,500 milligrams of glucosamine and 1,200 milligrams of chondroitin or a placebo for two months. The results for the glucosamine/chondroitin combination were promising.

Gelatin

Collagen forms the interlocking strands that help give cartilage its strength. It is a protein made up mainly of the amino acids glycine, proline, and hydroxyproline. Gelatin is an inexpensive animal protein that's rich in those same amino acids, which is why food giant Nabisco has dusted off its old Knox Gelatin, added some vitamin C and calcium, and is selling it as a new dietary supplement called NutraJoint.

What evidence does the maker of gelatin have to back up its claim that NutraJoint is "for everybody who wants to maintain flexible joints and healthy bones"? The only published study of gelatin in humans was completed in Czechoslovakia in 1985. Of fifty-one men and women with arthritis of the hips and knees who were given a daily dose of a gelatin similar to that in NutraJoint for two months, about half reported less pain (but no increase in mobility) compared with people who took a placebo. Gelatin is a supplement that you may want to try in order to see if it relieves your pain.

Vitamins C and D

Subjects in the Framingham Osteoarthritis Cohort Study underwent knee evaluations by radiography and dietary assessment via a questionnaire. Researchers found that a high intake of the antioxidant vitamins, especially vitamin C, may reduce the risk of cartilage loss as well as alleviate the progression of osteoarthritis. Furthermore, low intake and blood levels of vitamin D are associated with greater progression of osteoarthritis in the knee joint. Typical dosages of these vitamins are 500 to 1,000 milligrams of vitamin C per day and 400 IU of vitamin D per day.

SAMe

S-adenosylmethionine (SAMe) is a natural substance. The body man-ufactures it when the amino acid methionine is combined with ATP, the energy source in muscles. Because SAMe is a methyl donor (a carbon with three attached hydrogen atoms), it contributes sulfur molecules for rebuilding cell membranes, removing wastes and toxins, and making the mood-elevating neurotransmitters dopamine and serotonin. SAMe levels drop as we age and also drop in individuals with osteoarthritis, muscle pain, depression, and liver disease. In addition to its use as a supplement in alleviating depression, supplementing with SAMe has been shown to reduce osteoarthritis pain as effectively as ibuprofen, with fewer side ef-fects. SAMe is also considered an anti-inflammatory and pain reliever in hip and knee arthritis. SAMe even increases cartilage formation, while nonsteroidal anti-inflammatory drugs can actually accelerate cartilage damage.

Most experts recommend starting with 200 milligrams for a few days and working up to 400 milligrams three times per day after a few weeks.

MSM

Methylsulfonylmethane (MSM), an organic sulfur, has gained recog-nition for its ability to relieve inflammation and the resulting pain associ-ated with arthritis and other inflammation-related diseases affecting the muscles and joints. Clinical studies have shown that it can alleviate pain, reduce stiffness and swelling, and improve joint flexibility. In addition to decreasing inflammation, MSM is also known to promote blood flow, which helps the healing process, and to reduce painful muscle spasms.

One of the most significant applications of MSM is its demonstrated ability to alleviate pain associated with systemic inflammatory disorders. People with arthritis report substantial and long-lasting relief while sup-plementing MSM in their diet with daily dosages ranging from as low as 100 milligrams to as high as 5,000 milligrams. MSM's beneficial effect is due in part to its ability to sustain cell flow-through—that is, allowing harmful substances such as lactic acid to flow out while permitting nutrients to flow in, thereby preventing pressure buildup in cells that causes inflammation in the joints and elsewhere.

In one study, eight people suffering various forms of intractable pain were given MSM supplements in differing amounts for periods of up to nineteen months. All reported reduced levels of pain. If you are suffering from joint pain or swelling, you might want to try MSM, as well as glucosamine and chondroitin.

CONCLUSION

With age, many of us modify our training. The stretching and cross training that seemed a waste of time fifteen years ago may now be what allow us to continue to train consistently. Yet although we might acknowledge that increasing years merit changes in our training, we probably don't think the same about our diet. Masters athletes, however, can benefit from altering their menus along with their miles.

As we get older, we need more of some nutrients and less of others, and the number of calories needed decreases slightly. Unfortunately, there has been little research on how the nutritional needs of older athletes differ from those of their younger counterparts. The recommended daily allowances (RDAs) do not take into consideration the needs of more active persons, especially those over age fifty; it's assumed that everyone in that age group is sedentary. It's suggested that adjustments to nutrient intake be made according to one's level of activity. This is difficult, especially because aging causes the body's metabolic rate to decrease and its tendency to gain weight to increase.

So what's a rational, healthy masters athlete to do? Masters athletes are fortunate in that they can and should eat more nutritionally dense foods to obtain the vitamins and minerals they need. Eating healthy foods, training properly, and using proper supplementation for recovery can extend your training and add to an already long athletic career.

Nutrition for Every Day

Nutrition for performance is not just about what you eat directly before or after exercise to help you run faster, cycle harder, or extend your training session. Every day, you have to eat a selection of foods that supplies essential nutrients and energy just to carry out your day-to-day activities. As an athlete, you want to optimize your daily diet so that you have additional energy for exercise as well as the nutrients you need in order to aid your body's building and repair processes. This means that you have to eat more of the right foods, in specific proportions, to ensure good health and maximum performance.

There are six categories of nutrients that your body needs for survival. The four basic nutrients—also known as macronutrients—are water, carbohydrate, fat, and protein. The two remaining classes of nutrients are vitamins and minerals, which are discussed in Chapter 14. To ensure maximum performance, both in your everyday routine and in your training program, you need to include the healthiest forms of these nutrients in your diet. In addition, it's important to maintain the proper balance of macronutrients for your sport and activity level.

The unfortunate fact is that the typical American diet includes far too high a proportion of fat, sodium, and sugar. Although this kind of diet is adequate for everyday life, it's clearly not nutritious—that is, it doesn't provide your body with the right nutrients in the correct amounts for optimum health. What's more, an excess of high-fat, sugar-sweetened foods can lead to numerous health problems, including heart disease, diabetes, and certain types of cancer.

This chapter focuses on the four basic nutrients that are essential for optimal health and performance, paying particular attention to the energy-yielding nutrients carbohydrate, fat, and protein. The material provides general guidelines to help you include more of the "good" forms of these nutrients in your daily diet, not only to prevent disease but also to maintain overall good health.

WATER

Of the four basic nutrients, water is the most essential in maintaining life. Although it contains no energy in the form of calories, water is involved in almost every function of the body. Therefore, replacing water that is continuously lost through sweating and excretion is very important. While the body can survive for several weeks without food, it cannot survive for more than a few days without water.

As mentioned earlier, fluid intake should equal fluid loss. Because the typical 155-pound person loses about 2,300 milliliters (or 2.3 liters) of fluid per day, not including fluids lost from sweat during exercise, a comparable amount of fluid should be provided. The body obtains fluid mainly from fluids ingested, food consumed, and fluids produced by the body.

Approximately 60 percent of the fluid obtained by the body is from liquids that are consumed. The nutrients available in the different fluids vary quite substantially. For the most part, the only other nutrient obtained from water is fluoride if the water has been fluoridated. However, water is a very appropriate fluid when dehydration is to be combated. Some of the nutrients found in other fluids include calcium and vitamin D in milk, vitamin C in fruit juices, and tannins in tea, which can inhibit the absorption of iron. Overall, in recent years, the consumption of soft drinks, fruit juices, and fruit drinks has increased while the consumption of coffee, tea, and milk has decreased. Since the 1980s, the consumption of soft drinks has increased so much that more soft drinks are now consumed than milk and fruit juices combined.

Fluids from foods make up another 30 percent of the fluid obtained by the body. Some foods such as tomatoes, watermelon, and lettuce are very high in fluid content. Other foods such as cereal, nuts, and cookies contain much less fluid. Approximately 95 percent of the fluid obtained from food sources is absorbed by the body, with only a small amount remaining in the intestine and excreted by the body in the feces.

Many scientists recommend that fluid intake from food and drinks combined should be 1 to 1.5 milliliters per calorie expended, or approximately one quart per 1,000 calories expended. For people in caloric balance—that is, the calories expended equal the calories consumed—fluid intake can also be expressed as one quart per 1,000 calories consumed. However, for people who are dieting and consuming fewer calories than they are expending, the guidelines for fluid intake must use the calories expended to ensure proper hydration.

The body produces the remaining 10 percent of the fluid obtained by the body. During the metabolic breakdown of carbohydrate, lipids, or protein, water is an end product. As the total amount of water produced by the body is very small, generally between 150 to 250 milliliters per day, fluid must be consumed daily to maintain proper hydration levels.

CARBOHYDRATE

Carbohydrate is the body's primary energy source for all activities. Through digestion and metabolism, carbohydrate is broken down into glucose molecules, which can either be used for immediate energy or stored as glycogen. In previous chapters, we focused on stimulating insulin with carbohydrate and protein—in the proper ratio—to replenish glycogen rapidly. As you will remember, the first two hours after exercise are a period of maximum insulin sensitivity, when glycogen synthesis occurs at a faster-than-normal rate to give your body a "jump start" in replenishing glycogen. Your body continues to rebuild energy stores in the hours after, however, so it's important to optimize your carbohydrate intake during this time to ensure enough energy for school- or work-related activities and training sessions alike.

Optimizing carbohydrate intake means more than just consuming adequate amounts to replenish glycogen. Athletes also need to consider the types of carbohydrates they eat and when they eat them. For example, simple carbohydrates consist of monosaccharides, which are single sugar molecules. Monosaccharides such as glucose do not need to be broken down, and therefore, they enter the bloodstream immediately, providing a quick supply of energy. Simple carbohydrates, when consumed just before and during exercise, can maintain blood sugar for energy and spare glycogen. On the other hand, complex carbohydrates, including starch and glycogen, are composed of long chains of glucose molecules, known as polysaccharides. These chains have to be broken down before your body can use the glucose; therefore, complex carbohydrates provide your body with a steady supply of energy for a longer duration.

Fiber is a type of polysaccharide that your body cannot break down for energy. However, dietary fiber, which is also called *roughage*, helps the intestines to function efficiently and aids absorption of sugars into the bloodstream. Fiber-rich diets also promote a feeling of satiety, or fullness. In addition, research has shown that people who eat high-fiber diets experience reduced rates of cardiovascular disease, colon cancer, and diabetes.

Dietary Guidelines for Carbohydrate

For maximum performance, you should consume about 60 percent of your total daily calories from carbohydrate, keeping in mind that carbohydrate contains 4 calories per gram. For example, if your daily requirement is 2,400 calories, you would take in 1,440 calories from carbohydrate each day. To calculate your required carbohydrate intake, simply multiply your total daily calories by 0.60, or 60 percent. You can achieve roughly the same intake by consuming 3 to 5 grams of carbohydrate for every pound of your body weight. Again, that would be 3 grams per pound of body weight on easy days, 4 grams on moderate to hard days, and 5 grams on days when you're carbohydrate loading (see Chapter 16) or putting in a heavy endurance day.

When you choose carbohydrate-rich foods for your diet, try to select unrefined foods such as fruits, vegetables, peas, beans, pasta, and whole-grain products. It's wise to avoid processed foods, including soft drinks, desserts, candy, and sugar, which offer few, if any, of the vitamins and minerals that are important to your health. Another problem is that foods high in refined simple sugars are often high in fat, which should be limited in a healthy diet. Be aware that it's important not to skip meals, because this may lead to low blood glucose, which will in turn compromise protein and glycogen synthesis.

During my work with the National Cycling Team training camps at the Olympic Training Center in Colorado Springs, Colorado, I was surprised to find that many athletes did not know how to select high-carbohydrate foods. Often, the foods that athletes believe are high in carbohydrates are instead high in fat. Fortunately, there's an easy method for separating the high-carbohydrate foods from their imposters.

Let's assume, for example, that you choose a chocolate croissant for breakfast. One croissant (one serving) has 25 grams of carbohydrate and 260 calories per serving. You can calculate the percentage of carbohydrate in the croissant in two simple steps:

1. First, multiply the number of grams of carbohydrate per serving by four:

$$25 \times 4 = 100$$

   This gives you the total number of carbohydrate calories per serving.

2. Now, divide the number of carbohydrate calories by the total
   number of calories per serving:

$$100 \div 260 = .38, \text{ or } 38 \text{ percent}$$

As you can see above, your chocolate croissant is 38 percent carbohydrate. Clearly, this is not a high-carbohydrate food.

Sports Bars and Gels

Sports bars and gels are handy pre-exercise snacks. Many individuals eat irregularly or skip meals due to the time constraints
of work, social events, and training. When you forgo meals, however, your blood glucose drops and you're more likely to tire
sooner and feel lightheaded. Eating a high-carbohydrate snack an
hour or so before exercise will help to maintain your blood glucose
levels so that you can perform optimally. Michael Sherman, Ph.D.,
and colleagues at the Ohio State University in Columbus, found
that performance was improved by 12.5 percent when carbohydrate was consumed an hour before exercise. Try to consume 15 to
75 grams of carbohydrate in the hour before your workout.

The energy boost you get from eating a sports bar or gel before
or during exercise isn't due to the minor ingredients such as vitamins and minerals that some products contain. Instead, the carbohydrate in bars (about 23 to 47 grams) and gels (about 17 to 25
grams) elevates your blood glucose to provide energy for the exercising muscles.

Sports bars and gels are also an accessible energy source during
exercise. Consuming carbohydrate during workouts that last an
hour or more enables you to run longer and harder by providing

continued

glucose for your muscles when they're running out of carbohydrate. Thus, carbohydrate utilization (and therefore energy production) can continue at a high rate, and endurance is enhanced. Edward Coyle, Ph.D., at the University of Texas in Austin, has shown that consuming carbohydrate during exercise at 70 percent of maximum aerobic capacity can delay fatigue by thirty to sixty minutes. For the best results, try to take in 30 to 60 grams of carbohydrate (120 to 240 carbohydrate calories) for every hour of exercise. You can obtain this amount from either sports bars, gels, high-carbohydrate foods, or carbohydrate-containing sports drinks. Each carbohydrate form (solid, gel, or liquid) has advantages and drawbacks.

High-carbohydrate foods such as sports bars, fig bars, and fruit provide a feeling of satiety that you won't get from drinking fluids or sucking down gels. Sports bars and gels purposely have a very low water content so that they can be compact and easily carried. By comparison, high-carbohydrate foods that have high water content, such as fruit, take up more room. For example, to get the amount of carbohydrate supplied by one Power Bar (about 45 grams), you'd have to eat one and one-half bananas (45 grams). One gel packet supplies only slightly less carbohydrate (25 grams) than one banana (30 grams). And whereas bars and gels have a fairly long "shelf life," that banana may turn into black mush in your fanny pack within hours.

However, the low water content of sports bars and gels also has a downside. You'd better drink plenty of water (8 ounces) when you eat a sports bar before or during exercise. Otherwise, the product will settle poorly and you may feel there's a rock in your gut. Drink at least 4 ounces of water per gel packet or you will become nauseated. In addition to aiding your digestion, drinking water after consuming the bar or gel encourages you to hydrate

continued

adequately. Keep in mind that sports drinks containing 6 to 8 per cent carbohydrate (about 56 to 77 calories per 8 ounces) are a practical energy source for workouts lasting around an hour. Sports drinks provide the right proportion of water to carbohydrate to provide energy and replace fluid loss.

FAT

Lately, there has been a great deal of confusion concerning the place that fats have in the diet. Reports linking high-fat diets to illnesses such as heart disease, certain cancers, and diabetes have driven some people to reduce the fat in their diets to very low levels. However, studies have shown that this extreme can be unhealthy as well. Why? The fact is that some amount of dietary fat is essential for good health. Besides being your body's most concentrated source of energy, fat provides insulation and acts as protective padding for your bones and internal organs. And fats known as phospholipids are components of all cell membranes and other cellular structures, such as mitochondria.

A diet containing a moderate amount of fat is important for athletes who wish to maximize their performance and who need to increase their caloric consumption. Many athletes do not eat enough fat simply because they eat a high-carbohydrate diet, including more than 70 percent of calories from carbohydrate on a regular basis. In addition, some athletes are "fat phobic"—they cut back on their intake of fat because they have been led to believe that all fat is bad for their health. So while they train long and hard in an effort to stimulate their muscles' fat utilization, they often eat a diet depleted of fat, which sends the conflicting signal to their muscles that building extra machinery for metabolizing fat is a waste of cellular energy and space.

Unfortunately, the typical American diet includes too much total fat, too much of the wrong kinds of fats, and too little of the right kinds. The solution to this dietary dilemma, then, is not simply to cut fat out of your diet. Instead, it's important to have a working knowledge about some of the different types of fats and how they affect or are utilized by the body.

Fatty Acids

As we first discussed in Chapter 2, fats are composed of fatty acids. There are three major types of fatty acids found in the diet and in the body—saturated, polyunsaturated, and monounsaturated.

Saturated fatty acids tend to be solid at room temperature. They are found mainly in animal products, including whole milk, cream, cheese, and fatty meats. A diet high in saturated fat increases the amount of cholesterol circulating in the blood. Therefore, including too many saturated fats in the diet can significantly raise the blood cholesterol level, especially the level of the "bad" low-density lipoprotein (LDL) cholesterol.

Polyunsaturated fatty acids are generally liquid at room temperature and are found in corn, soybean, safflower, and sunflower oils. Although these fats have been shown to reduce total blood cholesterol level, they may also lower the level of the "good" high-density lipoprotein (HDL) cholesterol. Monounsaturated fatty acids, on the other hand, seem to lower LDL cholesterol without affecting HDL cholesterol. Olive, peanut, high-oleic sunflower, and canola oils have high amounts of monounsaturated fats.

In our bodies, dietary fatty acids are used as a source of chemical energy for our cells, second only to glucose in importance. Whereas some tissues, such as the brain, depend almost exclusively on glucose as an energy source, other tissues, notably the muscles, use fatty acids in addition to glucose. In fact, the most important muscle of all—the heart—normally gets about 60 percent of its energy from the metabolism of fatty acids.

Fatty acids that are not immediately used as an energy source are normally converted to fat molecules, which the body stores in its adipose tissues. Most fats and oils (oils are just fats in liquid form) consist of molecules called triglycerides. A triglyceride is composed of three fatty acid molecules linked to a molecule of glycerol (which is also a source of chemical energy). When the body needs to tap its fat reserves for energy, the triglycerides are broken down to their constituent fatty acids and glycerol.

ESSENTIAL FATTY ACIDS

Essential fatty acids (EFAs) are necessary for rebuilding and producing new cells, and for maintaining proper brain and nervous-system function. Although they are essential for health, EFAs cannot be made by the body—they must be obtained from the diet. Omega-3 and omega-6 fats are the two EFAs that we require for good health. Omitting these fatty acids from the diet can result in serious health problems.

Omega-3 fats, in particular, have been found to reduce the risk of heart disease and to lower blood pressure. The problem is that many of us don't include enough of the omega-3s in our diets. It's not that these EFAs don't occur naturally in a variety of foods. We just don't eat enough of the foods that are good sources of omega-3s, such as fresh deepwater fish, fish oil, and certain vegetable oils, including canola, flaxseed, and walnut oils.

In contrast to omega-3 fatty acids, the omega-6 fats are much more available. Omega-6 fats are found primarily in raw nuts, seeds, and legumes, and in unsaturated vegetable oils, such as grape seed oil, primrose oil, sesame oil, and soybean oil. They also occur in some amount in chicken, turkey, lamb, and pork. While no one knows the exact amount of omega-3 and omega-6 fats needed for optimal health, researchers are warning us to be careful to maintain a good balance of these EFAs. A healthy ratio is said to be no more than three times more omega-6 than omega-3 fatty acids. High levels of omega-6 fatty acids, out of balance with the omega-3s, can promote health problems such as heart disease, asthma, autoimmune diseases, diabetes, and weakened nerve fibers.

Dietary Guidelines for Fat

Because some amount of fat is necessary to maintain optimum health, your daily diet should include about 25 percent of calories from fat. Each gram of fat contains 9 calories, making it your body's most concentrated source of energy, with more than twice the energy of a gram of carbohydrate. To figure out your fat allowance, multiply your total calorie intake per day by 0.25, or 25 percent.

This level of fat intake represents approximately 45 to 55 grams per day for people who eat 2,000 calories per day, and 78 to 97 grams per day of fat for those consuming 3,500 calories per day. Many athletes who are trying to achieve a lean build consume less than 20 percent of energy from fat. They should be cautioned against consuming less than 15 percent of their energy from fat. This is especially true for people with a low energy intake—that is, those who eat fewer than 1,500 calories per day.

Research suggests that very low-fat diets (5 to 15 percent of energy from fat) do not provide additional health or performance benefits over a moderate fat diet and are usually very difficult to follow. In fact, athletes who keep their fat intakes at 20 to 25 percent of energy intake may find they feel better, are more successful in weight maintenance, and are less preoccupied with food. Active individuals attempting to eliminate fat from their diets frequently begin by eliminating meat, dairy products, eggs, and nuts.

In general, endurance athletes need to maintain higher levels of fat intake than do strength athletes. It's important to remember, however, that all athletes should focus on reducing their saturated-fat intake and on increasing their intake of the essential fatty acids, particularly the omega-3s. The following tips can help you to increase your EFA intake:

- Use olive and canola oils when cooking instead of margarine and butter.
- Aim to eat 3 to 9 ounces of fish a week.
- Use walnuts, almonds, and other nuts more frequently as a topping for cereal, yogurt, and salads.
- Add flaxseed oil to your diet.
- Select whole-grain products over refined versions for small amounts of essential fats.

As a general rule, you should try to avoid—or at least try to lower your intake of—whole-milk products, butter, egg yolks, cream cheese, and fatty meats such as bacon, hot dogs, bologna, and hamburgers. Coconut and palm oils, as well as organ meats, including kidney and liver, are also foods that you should eat only occasionally. These foods are all high in saturated fatty acids and cholesterol. Instead, eat lean meats such as fish, chicken, and turkey; egg whites; and skim-milk products.

Regarding sources of pure fat, such as oils, food sources high in polyunsaturated fats should be substituted for food sources high in saturated fats. Fat sources to avoid include butter, bacon fat, cream, mayonnaise, and mayonnaise-based salad dressings.

PROTEIN

So far, when we have discussed protein, it has been in terms of structural units called amino acids. Of the more than twenty amino acids that have been identified, nine have been identified as essential amino acids, meaning that the body cannot manufacture them. Essential amino acids, therefore, must be obtained from dietary sources. Complete proteins are proteins that contain all of the nine essential amino acids in sufficient amounts for adequate growth and development. Meat, fish, dairy products, and eggs have complete proteins.

Incomplete proteins are missing one or more of the essential amino acids, which negatively affects growth and developmental rates. However, your body can actually manufacture complete proteins if you consume a variety of plant foods, such as beans, grains, vegetables, fruits, nuts, and seeds, that contain essential amino acids, as well as sufficient calories every day. This is good news for vegetarians, who do not eat animal foods to obtain complete proteins. Evidence even suggests that well-balanced vegetarian meals may decrease the risk of heart disease and cancer, because they're lower in fat and higher in complex carbohydrates than the typical American diet.

Dietary Guidelines for Protein

You should aim to consume about 15 to 20 percent of your total calorie intake from protein. Simply multiply your daily caloric intake by 0.15, or 15 percent, to calculate your protein requirement. Therefore, if you take in 2,400 calories per day, 360 of those calories should come from protein. As with carbohydrate, protein has about 4 calories per gram.

When you calculate your protein requirement, remember to take into consideration the duration and intensity of your activity. Some types of exercise require athletes to consume more calories from protein. Athletes who exercise for several hours at a time can actually lose muscle mass because they burn a high percentage of protein for fuel. To help maintain muscle mass, these athletes may benefit from up to 0.85 gram of protein for every pound of body weight.

Based on current research findings, ranges for endurance athletes for protein intake per day are:

- Moderate training (about sixty minutes per day): about 0.6 to 0.7 gram per pound.
- Moderately hard training: about 0.7 to 0.85 gram per pound.
- Heavy, long, hard training: about 0.85 gram per pound.

One of the challenges with protein intake is to choose protein sources that are healthy and complete. Animal foods, such as dairy products, meat, and eggs, provide all the essential amino acids that you need to build and develop muscle. However, these foods can add an unhealthy amount of the wrong kinds of fats to your diet. A diet loaded with fat is an *atherogenic* diet, meaning that it increases your risk for heart disease. Your best bet, then, is to choose lean meats, such as poultry and lean red meat from which the fat has been trimmed; low-fat dairy products, including low-fat or skim milk; and most fishes and shellfishes. Remember that including more fish in your diet will also help you to boost your intake of the essential fatty acids.

Foods derived from plants, such as fruits, vegetables, and grains, are typically low in fat and cholesterol. Unfortunately, unlike animal proteins, plant proteins are generally incomplete in their essential–amino-acid content. It's possible to get an adequate balance of these amino acids, however, by combining different plant proteins. Eating fruits, vegetables, and grains in the proper combinations will enable you to get all of the amino acids you need to build muscle, without adding as much fat as animal proteins. A popular grain-and-vegetable combination is brown rice and corn. Peas and carrots are a good combination for complete proteins from legumes and vegetables. And even a peanut butter sandwich is sufficient for a grain-and-legume complete-protein combination.

Protein Supplements

In order to maintain muscle mass, athletes need to take in adequate protein to offset some of what is broken down for energy during exercise. This is not always easy. In fact, it's not uncommon for certain types of athletes, such as endurance athletes and weightlifters, to have difficulty consuming enough quality protein to meet their daily requirements, and this may not be from lack of trying! For athletes who require large quantities of protein daily, including these amounts in the diet may be a challenge. In these cases, a protein supplement may be just the answer.

If you think that you need to give your dietary protein intake a supplemental boost, keep in mind that protein consumed in excess is not converted to muscle. Instead, it's often converted to fat. Therefore, you should take special care to eat just the right amount for your weight and activity level.

MEAL-REPLACEMENT POWDERS

If you need extra protein, you may benefit from the convenience of a meal-replacement powder (MRP). These products are available in a wide array of flavors and nutrient combinations. The important thing to remember is to choose a supplement that's healthy and low in fat. A complete product should contain simple and complex carbohydrates and all of the essential amino acids. Use your supplement strategically to enhance rather than overwhelm your diet and recovery.

MRPs are typically low in calories (about 200 to 300 per serving) unless they are designed specifically for weight gain, and then some of the products are nearly 500 calories per serving. They generally contain a balance of high levels of protein (about 25 to 45 grams) and carbohydrate (about 15 to 30 grams) and a small amount of fat. They also have between 50 and 100 percent of the RDAs for many vital nutrients.

When MRPs started gaining widespread popularity in the early 1990s, there was a lot of hype and hyperbole, but the manufacturers didn't provide much, if any, scientific evidence to back it up. And sometimes, companies would refer to research findings that were extrapolated inappropriately. But that began to change, and research is beginning to appear on the benefits of MRPs.

Richard Kreider, Ph.D., FACSM, with the Exercise and Sport Nutrition Laboratory, Baylor University, conducted a study that looked at the effects of meal-replacement powders on football players. During eighty-four days of winter training and spring practice, about sixty players supplemented their diets with either a carbohydrate placebo or a typical, balanced-nutrient MRP that also contained creatine. Results indicated that average gains in lean mass were significantly greater in the MRP group than in the carbohydrate group.

MRPs provide a useful way to consume high levels of high-quality protein without the saturated fat that often accompanies traditional protein-rich foods. Different products contain different protein sources, some of which may be better absorbed by the body than others.

The amount of fat that is added to MRPs is minimal; it ranges from about 1 gram to 3 grams. But manufacturers use different types of fat and like to extol the benefits of their own special formula or gleefully point to the failings of a competitor's product.

Whether powdered food is for you depends on your goals and your nutritional habits. "I think they're mainly intended for the active person who can't eat as ideally as they'd like to," Kreider says.

By substituting a possibly high-calorie, high-fat meal with an MRP and maybe a piece of fruit, people can lower their calorie intake and eat a healthier diet. "We also have people who use these after they work out, and they feel their appetite is kind of reduced, so they don't eat as much later," he adds. "This is something you could use as a snack."

Investigating the 40-30-30 Diet

The 40-30-30 diet has recently become a popular nutritional regimen in the sports and fitness worlds. Athletes on this diet plan obtain 40 percent of their calories from carbohydrate, 30 percent from fat, and 30 percent from protein, in contrast to the 60-25-15 ratio that has traditionally been recommended by nutritionists. Supporters of the 40-30-30 plan say that decreasing carbohydrate intake and boosting protein consumption will enable dieters to burn more fat. For athletes, this translates into a glycogen-sparing effect, which can extend endurance.

The theory behind the 40-30-30 diet is that a lower carbohydrate intake coupled with an increased percentage of protein will help to keep insulin levels low in the blood. From what you've already learned about insulin's importance in glycogen manufacture and storage, you might be wondering what benefits low insulin levels would offer. While insulin is essential for processing carbohydrate, it has also been shown to inhibit fat metabolism. According to 40-30-30 proponents, lowering blood-insulin levels will allow the body to burn fat more efficiently.

Furthermore, whereas a high-carbohydrate, low-fat meal triggers the release of insulin, a higher percentage of protein will trigger the release of glucagon. This hormone has the opposite effect

continued

of insulin: it enables the body to burn fat. Therefore, in theory, an athlete who is looking to use more fat for energy during exercise would want to eat less carbohydrate and more protein and fat.

Many researchers in sports nutrition, however, have stated otherwise. The fact remains that the consumption of any moderate meal consisting of 60 percent of calories from carbohydrate, 25 percent from fat, and 15 percent from protein will produce a moderate amount of insulin. The primary role of insulin is to metabolize carbohydrate—not to store fat. Since insulin is busy doing its job on a carbohydrate-rich meal, the concentration of insulin soon falls.

The claim that the 40-30-30 diet helps athletes to lose body fat also remains unproven. It may be that those who lose body fat have done so not because 40-30-30 keeps insulin low in the blood but because they've benefited from calorie counting to stay within the recommended 2,000-calorie limit of the 40-30-30 diet. An athlete following this plan ends up eating less simply because he or she is taking greater care to count calories and to regulate food consumption.

In the end, most nutrition researchers, sports dietitians, and exercise physiologists remain firm in their conviction that the optimal athletic diet consists of 60 percent of calories from carbohydrate, 25 percent from fat, and 15 percent from protein. This recommendation is based on a veritable mountain of validated and convincing research. The experts also advocate supplementing with carbohydrate before and during exercise to improve endurance performance and consuming carbohydrate after exercise to replenish glycogen stores.

WHEY PROTEIN

Whey protein, once thought to be a useless byproduct of cheese production, has recently become one of the most popular protein supplements. This is due, in part, to the development of several methods for distilling whey into a high-quality powder that is fat and lactose free. Although it's the most expensive of the three protein powders (whey, casein, and soy), whey has a number of advantages over other protein supplements.

One of the greatest benefits of whey protein is that it enhances glutathione production. As you may remember from Chapter 8, glutathione is one of the body's natural antioxidants. Therefore, in addition to supplying protein, whey can help to protect against free-radical damage. Whey protein also has the highest levels of branched-chain amino acids (BCAAs), and it has been shown to boost the immune system. And because whey protein exits the stomach much faster than proteins such as casein, it can be absorbed more quickly into the bloodstream through the intestines. This provides a substantial rise in blood amino acids in a short amount of time, which is important during exercise and recovery. Finally, whey protein dissolves easily in water, making it convenient for a protein drink when you're on the go.

Whey protein contains the highest concentration (about 25 percent) of BCAAs of any single protein source. This BCAA content is important because BCAAs are an integral part of muscle development and are the first amino acids sacrificed to provide energy during high-intensity exercise.

Whey-protein isolate contains quadra-peptides (short protein chains containing four amino acids), which have been shown to have painkilling effects. This is another powerful functional property that may help decrease muscle soreness following intense weight training or aerobic exercise.

Due to its excellent amino-acid profile, solubility, and digestibility, whey has a high biological value (BV). Basically, BV is a measure of how well a protein is used by the body.

One of the more interesting properties of whey protein is its reported ability to stimulate IGF-1 (insulin-like growth factor 1) production. IGF-1 is structurally and functionally similar to insulin and enhances protein synthesis and increased muscle growth. Researchers have discovered that whey protein provides unique health benefits, such as fighting infections and perhaps even fighting cancer. Lastly, whey protein appears to play a direct role in bone growth. Studies show it may increase the level of bone proteins such as collagen and strengthen the bones.

Properly processed whey protein is the ideal protein for several reasons. Compared to casein, whey protein is digested more quickly, with better mixing characteristics and a general reputation for higher quality. It offers the highest content of BCAAs (more than 20 percent). This versatile protein can be used for baking, cooking, mixing shakes, and so on. It is ideal for both hard-training athletes and sedentary people who want to supplement their diets with more protein. Because of its high BV, less is needed to accomplish tissue repair, growth, and recovery. There are many excellent protein products on the market that contain only whey protein.

Casein

Casein, another byproduct of cheese production, is included in milk protein powders in varying proportions. Although casein has a higher glutamine content than whey protein, it contains fewer BCAAs. One disadvantage of milk protein powders is that they don't dissolve easily, so you'll probably need a blender to make your protein drinks. Another concern for some athletes is that casein contains lactose, or milk sugar, which some individuals are unable to digest. Lactose-containing products may cause some people to experience abdominal pain, diarrhea, and excessive gas.

One of the best uses of casein is as a drink before bed to lower muscle breakdown during sleep; it is also good for breakfast, to provide a steady stream of amino acids in the morning.

Soy Protein

Soy protein, which is high in BCAAs and glutamine, was the first type of protein powder on the market. The isoflavones (plant hormones, also called *phytoestrogens*) in this lower quality source of protein has been found to exert an estrogenic effect, which can be counterproductive for male athletes. For female athletes, however, the mild estrogenic activity may be beneficial. This is because soy isoflavones can ease menopausal symptoms and promote bone density and other positive effects of estrogen. A disadvantage of soy protein for both men and women is that it is low in methionine, an essential amino acid. Also, some people don't like the taste of soy products.

This protein is great for a dieting phase and can be used by anyone to improve general health. Many soy products require a blender, although newer, top-of-the-line products are easier to mix.

CONCLUSION

Above all else, balanced nutrition is paramount to your success as an athlete because it is crucial to your overall health. Every day, carbohydrate, fat, and protein supply you with energy for your daily activities and help your body to maintain and rebuild tissues. To ensure an adequate intake of these macronutrients, you should consume about 60 percent of calories from carbohydrate, 25 percent from fat, and 15 to 20 percent from protein.

Poor nutrition is a nationwide problem. The typical diet, even for active, health-conscious people, often consists of too much saturated fat and a high percentage of simple sugars. On the whole, we need to focus on increasing our intake of the "good" essential fatty acids while decreasing our intake of processed foods that are high in sugar and low in essential nutrients.

It's important to note that what's considered adequate nutrition for the nonathlete is most likely not adequate to meet your body's requirements. As an active person, you have increased energy needs, so you need to eat more of the energy-yielding macronutrients in the right proportions. You will also want to pay close attention to your protein intake, so that you can counteract some of the protein breakdown that occurs during exercise. This may require you to include a protein supplement in your diet in order to meet your elevated requirements.

Vitamins and Minerals:
Keys to Improved Performance

Micronutrients are nutrients that are found in the diet and in the body in small amounts. Although we only need trace amounts of these vitamins and minerals, they are essential for optimal performance and, more important, for overall good health. That's because micronutrients often act as *cofactors*, which must be present for other substances in the body to perform their numerous and diverse functions. As cofactors, these nutrients are involved in energy production, oxygen transport, muscle action, and growth. They are also important structural components in your body. And, as you learned in Chapter 8, some vitamins and minerals can act as antioxidants to protect your body from free-radical damage.

Ideally, our diets should supply all of the nutrients we need to meet our daily requirements. But in the real world, although we eat some amount of carbohydrate, fat, protein, and vitamins and minerals every day, the food we consume does not necessarily promote good health. Today, too many of us consume a high percentage of nutrient-poor processed foods that have lost some of their vitamins and minerals through factors such as freezing, shipping, and storage. Diets that include too much of these foods do not provide the nourishment necessary for optimum health. Instead, they supply the bare minimum of nutrients necessary for survival.

When you exercise, your energy needs increase. Inadequate nutrition combined with the physical stress of exercise—on top of life's everyday stresses—may be enough to cause a deficiency of one or several important vitamins and minerals. Therefore, even a diet that is considered to be optimal for a more sedentary person will not be adequate to meet your elevated needs. Like many other athletes, you may find that you benefit from nutritional supplementation.

So how do you know if you are getting enough of the essential vitamins and minerals to ensure your well-being? The tendency in the past has been to base the definition of good health on the absence of disease. Clearly, this interpretation is not adequate guidance for the average American, so it's certainly not suitable for an athlete's needs. This chapter begins with a brief outline of the evolution of nutritional guidelines, from the now-outmoded Recommended Dietary Allowances (RDAs) to the most recent recommendations for athletes, known as the Performance Daily Intakes (PDIs). You will also find a comprehensive overview of the essential vitamins and minerals that your body requires—not just to prevent deficiency diseases but also to maintain optimum health.

A NEW STANDARD FOR SPORTS NUTRITION

Almost sixty years ago, the National Research Council (NRC) of the U.S. Department of Health and Human Services recognized the importance of establishing nutritional guidelines for good health. As a result, the Recommended Dietary Allowances (RDAs) were established as the standard for nutrition. In the years following, the NRC periodically published updated RDAs, based upon increasing evidence about nutrient allowances for maintaining health.

One of the problems with the RDAs was complexity: For each nutrient, separate recommendations were made based on gender, age, and other factors. By the mid-1980s, scientists and nutritionists disagreed so widely on the recommended allowances that an update was not published for several years. Finally, in 1993, the Nutrition Labeling and Education Act replaced the RDAs with the Reference Daily Intakes (RDIs), which gives the average recommendations for twenty-seven vitamins and minerals. By 1997, the RDIs had replaced the RDAs entirely.

The Reference Daily Intakes are not without their own problems, however. For example, like the RDAs, the RDIs represent allowances that are necessary to prevent deficiency. In other words, the RDIs recommend values for essential nutrition for survival—they are not recommendations for amounts that will promote optimum health.

In truth, our bodies need higher amounts of nutrients than the RDIs recommend. Nutritionists such as Shari Lieberman, Ph.D., coauthor of *The Real Vitamin and Mineral Book,* have revolutionized the science of nutrition by establishing new guidelines called Optimum Daily Intakes (ODIs). These are recommendations for higher allowances of the vitamins and minerals that we require for physical well-being. They take into account the environmental stresses that we encounter every day, as well as the fact that we often don't meet our nutrient requirements through diet alone.

While nonathletes can maintain optimum health by eating balanced meals and supplementing according to the ODI recommendations, athletes must eat a diet that is much more complex. Dr. Kenneth Cooper, a groundbreaker in preventive medicine, recognized this need. In *Antioxidant Revolution,* Dr. Cooper addresses the need for active people to consume higher amounts of particular vitamins and minerals for protection from serious illnesses.

To help you ensure that you are meeting your requirements for optimum health and maximum athletic performance, I suggest that you follow a new set of standards called the Performance Daily Intakes (PDIs).

These guidelines were first presented by Daniel Gastelu, M.S., M.F.S., and Fred Hatfield, Ph.D., in their book *Dynamic Nutrition for Maximum Performance*. The PDIs are guidelines for physically active men and women that compensate for the higher nutritional requirements that athletes have over nonathletes.

The remaining sections of this chapter detail the functions and dietary sources of the individual vitamins and minerals. For each nutrient, I have included the recommended Performance Daily Intake, according to the most recent research on the connection between nutrition and performance.

WHAT ARE VITAMINS?

Vitamins are organic compounds that regulate and facilitate the millions of chemical reactions that take place in your body. They do not provide your body with energy in and of themselves, but they do play a role in breaking down and releasing energy from the macronutrients carbohydrate, fat, and protein. Your body cannot make most vitamins, or at least not in substantial amounts, so you have to obtain them from foods or supplements.

The thirteen essential vitamins are divided into two groups. One group consists of fat-soluble vitamins, which the body is capable of storing for weeks or months in the fatty portions of body tissues. The second group consists of water-soluble vitamins, which are found in your body's fluids; these need to be replenished daily because they are rapidly excreted.

The Fat-Soluble Vitamins

Vitamins A, D, E, and K are fat-soluble vitamins that are stored in the liver and fatty tissues until the body needs them. These nutrients require the presence of fats in the diet to be properly digested and absorbed. Therefore, deficiencies are generally reported in individuals who consume diets that are extremely low in fat. Be aware, however, that you need to be especially careful when you supplement with any of these vitamins: When consumed in excess, they have the potential to reach harmful levels in the body because of their storage capabilities.

VITAMIN A

Vitamin A is well known for its effectiveness in promoting clear vision and preventing night blindness. It is also needed for cellular growth and development, and for maintaining and repairing all epithelial tissues, which make up the skin and internal linings of the respiratory and digestive tracts. Vitamin A functions in the formation of bones and teeth, and it helps to support the immune system as well. Good sources of vitamin A include liver, fish-liver oil, egg yolks, crab, halibut, whole-milk products, butter, cream, and margarine.

Carotenoids are chemicals found in yellow-red plant pigments that can be chemically converted into vitamin A in the body. The best known of the carotenoids is beta-carotene, which functions as an antioxidant to neutralize free radicals and prevent oxidative damage. Carrots, green leafy vegetables, spinach, broccoli, squash, apricots, sweet potatoes, and cantaloupe are foods rich in beta-carotene.

The PDI of vitamin A is 5,000 to 25,000 IU. For beta-carotene, the PDI is 15,000 to 60,000 IU for athletes who do not engage in endurance exercise, and 20,000 to 80,000 IU for endurance athletes.

VITAMIN D

Vitamin D supports bone formation and maintenance by aiding the body in absorbing calcium and phosphorus, two major structural components of bone tissue. Because of this function, it acts as insurance against rickets, a childhood disease that is characterized by soft, malformed bones, as well as osteoporosis. Vitamin D is believed to improve muscular strength and to enhance immunity, in addition to helping regulate heartbeat.

Vitamin D is found in foods such as eggs, butter, cream, and liver, and also in seafood, including halibut, herring, mackerel, salmon, sardines, and shrimp. Milk fortified with vitamin D is also a major dietary source.

The PDI of vitamin D is 400 to 1,000 IU.

VITAMIN E

As you will remember from Chapter 8, vitamin E is an antioxidant that is important in minimizing free-radical damage. It is also well known for its role in healing wounds because it is a component for normal blood clotting and tissue repair. The maintenance of healthy nerves is another one of vitamin E's many functions.

Dietary sources of vitamin E include soy, corn, cottonseed, peanut, and safflower oils. Vitamin E can also be found in sufficient amounts in dark green leafy vegetables, legumes, nuts, seeds, and whole grains.

The PDI of vitamin E is 200 to 1,000 IU.

VITAMIN K

Vitamin K is essential because it aids in the synthesis of *prothrombin*, a substance that is necessary for blood to clot. The body also uses this nutrient to produce *osteocalcin*, a protein found in large amounts only in bone, and from which calcium is made. Deficiencies of this vitamin are rarely reported because it can be manufactured by the "friendly" bacteria that inhabit the intestines.

The richest sources of vitamin K include green leafy vegetables, asparagus, blackstrap molasses, broccoli, and cabbage. Milk and other dairy products, eggs, cereal, and fruits contain small amounts of vitamin K.

The PDI of vitamin K is 80 to 180 micrograms (mcg).

The Water-Soluble Vitamins

Vitamins B_1 (thiamine), B_2 (riboflavin), B_3 (niacin), B_5 (pantothenic acid), B_6 (pyridoxine), B_{12} (cobalamin), and C, as well as folate and biotin, are all water-soluble vitamins. The body absorbs these nutrients easily, but because they are quickly excreted in the urine, they are not stored in any significant amount. For this reason, it's important to make sure that you get adequate amounts of the water-soluble vitamins on a daily basis.

VITAMIN B COMPLEX

The B-complex family of vitamins includes all of the B vitamins plus folate and biotin. These vitamins are important *coenzymes*, which are cofactors that enable enzymes to carry out their important functions. They help the body to use the macronutrients carbohydrate, fat, and protein to produce energy. Vitamin B_6 functions to help the body use amino acids to manufacture proteins, which are then incorporated into body tissues, used to make hormones, or metabolized for energy. Both vitamin B_{12} and folate aid in cell multiplication and are necessary for the synthesis of red blood cells, which carry oxygen to other body cells.

Table 14.1 below summarizes some of the sources of the B vitamins, as well as the Performance Daily Intake for each vitamin in the B-complex family.

Table 14.1. Sources of B-Complex Vitamins

B-COMPLEX VITAMIN	SOURCES	PERFORMANCE DAILY INTAKE
B_1 (thiamine)	beans, brewer's yeast, peanuts, peas, pork, organ meats, wheat germ	30–200 mg
B_2 (riboflavin)	brewer's yeast, dairy products, fish, fortified grain products, green vegetables, meat, nuts, poultry	30–200 mg
B_3 (niacin)	brewer's yeast, lean meats, legumes, liver, nuts, potatoes, whole grains	20–100 mg
B_5 (pantothenic acid)	beef, eggs, fish, most fruits and vegetables, milk, pork, potatoes, whole wheat	25–200 mg
B_6 (pyridoxine)	bananas, chicken, eggs, fish, kidney, liver, peanuts, brown rice, soybeans, walnuts	20–100 mg
B_{12} (cobalamin)	beef, clams, eggs, herring, lamb, mackerel, oysters, poultry, tofu	12–200 mcg

B-COMPLEX VITAMIN	SOURCES	PERFORMANCE DAILY INTAKE
Biotin	asparagus, beef, brewer's yeast, eggs, green leafy vegetables, lamb, pork, salmon, whole wheat	125–250 mcg
Folate	brewer's yeast, cauliflower, cereal, egg yolks, legumes, liver, milk, nuts, soy flour	400–1,000 mcg

VITAMIN C

Vitamin C (ascorbic acid) is probably best known for its role in preventing the common cold and in fighting infections. However, it is also required for the production and maintenance of collagen, which is a component of bones, teeth, skin, and tendons. Therefore, it's an important nutrient for the healing of wounds and burns. As an antioxidant, vitamin C helps to minimize free-radical damage.

Because the body cannot manufacture vitamin C, it must be obtained from dietary sources or in the form of supplements. Therefore, ensuring adequate intake is very important. Good food sources include citrus fruits, strawberries, tomatoes, potatoes, and vegetables such as green and red peppers, broccoli, Brussels sprouts, collard greens, and spinach.

The PDI of vitamin C is 800 to 3,000 milligrams.

WHAT ARE MINERALS?

Minerals are *inorganic* nutrients, or nutrients that are not derived from plant or animal matter. They come from the earth's surface and are absorbed by plants through their roots and incorporated into the structure of the plants. We eventually eat the plants or the animals that eat plants, and the minerals become part of our own body structure.

Every living cell on this planet depends upon minerals for proper function and structure. Minerals are essential for muscle contraction and the maintenance of healthy nerve function. They also regulate fluid balance, transport substances throughout the body, aid in the formation of bones and blood, and help maintain muscle tone. Like vitamins, minerals enable your body to perform its functions—including energy production—repeatedly and at lightning speed.

Because they are contained in different amounts in the body, minerals are classified according to two groups: the major, or *macro*, minerals; and the trace, or *micro*, minerals. Major minerals are required and contained in your body in larger amounts than are trace minerals. However, both major and trace minerals can cause toxic side effects when they are taken in excessive amounts. Therefore, you should supplement with minerals according to the recommended guidelines and avoid experimenting with doses that exceed your suggested daily intake.

Major Minerals

The major minerals include calcium, magnesium, phosphorus, and sulfur, as well as the electrolytes chloride, potassium, and sodium. Although magnesium can also function as an electrolyte, it has many non-electrolyte functions, which we will address specifically in this section.

Major minerals are generally found in the body in amounts larger than 5 grams. Because they are present in larger total quantities, the major minerals influence the body fluids, thereby affecting the whole body in a general way.

CALCIUM

Calcium is an essential mineral for healthy bone formation and maintenance. In fact, 99 percent of the body's calcium is contained in the bones of the skeleton as calcium phosphate. The other 1 percent circulates in blood and other body fluids and is contained in the body's soft tissues.

Calcium's diverse roles in the body are not limited to the upkeep of bone tissue. For example, calcium is necessary for muscle growth, as well as for the contraction and relaxation of muscles—including the heart. Calcium is also involved in nerve-impulse transmission and blood clotting.

Many of us automatically think of dairy products such as milk, cheese, ice cream, sour cream, cottage cheese, and yogurt as being high in calcium. However, broccoli, kale, collard greens, oysters, shrimp, salmon, and clams are also good sources of calcium that should not be overlooked.

The PDI of calcium is 1,200 to 2,600 milligrams daily.

Special Considerations for Women. Because exercise is known to strengthen existing bone and stimulate the formation of new bone, it is often recommended for women who need to increase bone mass. However, it has been proven that strenuous or long-term exercise can actually have a negative effect on bone density. Surprisingly, increasing numbers of young women athletes actually suffer from a loss of bone mass or thinning of the bone, known as *osteoporosis.*

As it turns out, many women who exercise to "lose the fat" may unknowingly lower their body fat to unhealthy levels, below the suggested healthy level of at least 10 percent. Abnormally low body fat interferes with production of the hormone *estrogen*, which can result in the cessation of menstruation, known as *amenorrhea.* And because estrogen is also important in shifting calcium from the bloodstream into the bones, diminished estrogen levels cause the absorption of calcium by the bones to diminish. The end result is that the bones begin to weaken and gradually become brittle.

Unfortunately, simply supplementing with calcium is not the answer to this problem. The bones can only properly absorb calcium when it is in balance with other vitamins and minerals—especially magnesium. In fact, too much calcium can lead to magnesium deficiency. Therefore, women athletes who need to supplement with calcium should take magnesium along with calcium in the proper ratio. Most nutritionists now recommend that the calcium-to-magnesium ratio should be about 2 to 1. Women should also pay particular attention to their intake of several other bone-building nutrients, including vitamins C, D, and K, boron, manganese, and zinc.

MAGNESIUM

In Chapter 6, you learned how magnesium can function as an electrolyte in the body. But magnesium serves many purposes apart from its role as an electrolyte. It is a necessary element in hundreds of enzyme operations, including ATP production for energy. Magnesium also helps to form bones and teeth, and it aids in the uptake and balance of two essential minerals for bone development and maintenance—calcium and phosphorus. Researchers have speculated that moderate supplementation with magnesium has the potential to improve endurance and strength for performance. Unfortunately, athletes—in particular, those involved in endurance activities—tend to deplete their magnesium stores, most likely because the body's demand for magnesium increases with an increase in physical activity. Therefore, anyone who exercises would be wise to carefully monitor his or her magnesium intake.

Magnesium can be obtained from dietary sources such as apples, avocados, bananas, brown rice, dairy foods, garlic, green leafy vegetables, legumes, nuts, soybeans, and whole grains.

The PDI of magnesium is 400 to 800 milligrams.

Special Considerations for Women. Women athletes who supplement with calcium in an effort to prevent bone loss are strongly cautioned to monitor their magnesium intake. Remember that calcium and magnesium must be taken in the 2-to-1 ratio to work effectively. When the ratio is exceeded in favor of calcium, magnesium deficiency can sometimes result. This is because increased levels of calcium increase the demand for magnesium to aid in calcium uptake by the bones.

PHOSPHORUS

After calcium, phosphorus is the second most abundant mineral in the human body. Phosphorus is present in bone as part of calcium phosphate. It is also a component of both adenosine phosphate and creatine phosphate, which store the body's chemical energy. As a constituent of membrane phospholipids, phosphorus functions in maintaining cell membranes as well. The metabolism of fat and carbohydrate also depends, in part, on the presence of phosphorus.

The best sources of phosphorus are milk, fish, eggs, asparagus, bran, brewer's yeast, corn, legumes, nuts, meats, poultry, and salmon; and sesame, sunflower, and pumpkin seeds.

The PDI of phosphorus is 800 to 1,600 milligrams.

SULFUR

Sulfur is part of the chemical structure of many amino acids, including methionine and glutathione. It is found in hemoglobin and in all body tissues, and it is needed for the synthesis of collagen. Sulfur also helps to disinfect the blood, and it aids in the body's defenses against toxic substances.

Food sources of sulfur include Brussels sprouts, dried beans, cabbage, eggs, fish, garlic, meats, onions, and soybeans.

A PDI has not yet been established for sulfur.

ELECTROLYTES

As we discussed earlier in the book, electrolytes are minerals—including sodium, chloride, and potassium—that conduct the electrical energy of the body and regulate the flow of water between the cells and the bloodstream. (See page 190 for a discussion of magnesium.) Sodium and chloride are contained mainly in the body's *extracellular fluids*, which are any fluids that are found in the areas of the body outside the cells. Blood and lymph are extracellular fluids. Potassium, on the other hand, is the body's primary electrolyte that is contained in *intracellular fluid*, meaning fluid that is found within cells. For a more detailed discussion of the body's major electrolytes, refer to Chapter 6.

The PDI of both sodium and chloride is 1,500 to 4,500 milligrams. The PDI of potassium is 2,500 to 4,000 milligrams.

Trace Minerals

The trace minerals include boron, chromium, copper, iodine, iron, manganese, molybdenum, selenium, and zinc. These nutrients occur in the body in smaller amounts than do the major minerals, but they are no less important to our survival. Therefore, consistent intake is important.

BORON

Boron is a trace mineral that's essential for metabolizing calcium, phosphorus, and magnesium, and is therefore important for healthy bone formation. Although some researchers have speculated that boron can increase testosterone production, more research is needed to determine what other benefits it may hold for athletes.

Boron is found in leafy vegetables, fruit, nuts, and legumes. The PDI of boron is 5 to 10 milligrams.

CHROMIUM

Chromium aids insulin in the uptake of glucose by muscle cells for energy release. For this reason, a deficiency may result in high blood glucose. There is also evidence that chromium may help lower cholesterol. Furthermore, in the last several years, chromium has received widespread attention as a muscle-builder and fat-burner. Continuing research is necessary before scientists can draw any definite conclusions.

The food sources of chromium include black pepper, brewer's yeast, brown rice, cheese, liver, meat, mushrooms, nuts, potatoes, and whole grains. Chromium is easily processed out of foods, however, so people who eat diets high in refined foods are at risk for chromium deficiency. The PDI of chromium is 200 to 400 micrograms.

COPPER

Copper is an important trace mineral for the formation of hemoglobin, the compound in red blood cells that enables them to carry oxygen from the lungs to the tissues via the bloodstream. Collagen requires copper for proper formation as well. Copper is also present in many enzymes and is part of the body's natural antioxidant, superoxide dismutase, which helps to protect the body against free-radical damage. Copper has also attracted attention in the sports world for its role in the release of energy.

Nuts, seafood, chocolate, meat, mushrooms, and organ meats—especially liver—are all rich sources of copper. The PDI of copper is 3 to 6 milligrams.

IODINE

Iodine is required for the proper functioning of a gland located in the neck called the *thyroid gland*, which helps regulate metabolism, energy production, growth, and overall physical performance. Iodine deficiency can result in the enlargement of the thyroid, as the cells of the thyroid enlarge to trap as much iodine as possible. The enlargement of the thyroid gland sometimes becomes visible as a lump, which is known as a *goiter.*

Seafood is an excellent source of iodine. Other sources of iodine include iodized salt, spinach, meat, and dairy products. The iodine content of these foods varies depending on the content of the soil in which the plants were grown or off which animals grazed.

The PDI of iodine is 200 to 400 micrograms.

IRON

Iron is an essential mineral, necessary for the formation of the oxygen-carrying compounds *hemoglobin* and *myoglobin*. Hemoglobin ferries oxygen from the lungs to the tissues, and myoglobin carries oxygen within cells. Iron deficiency can result in decreased levels of hemoglobin or myoglobin, which will impair oxygen transport and ultimately limit athletic performance. When iron intake is low, the body depletes its stores in the bone marrow, spleen, and liver, which can result in the development of anemia.

Iron deficiency can also result from exercise. One possible route for iron loss is foot-strike hemolysis. This occurs because some red blood cells are destroyed when the soles of the feet make contact with the hard ground surface. In addition, exercise may cause small blood losses through the digestive tract, at least in some athletes.

Sports anemia is a temporary condition resulting from exercise. Early in training, blood plasma volume increases, which artificially lowers hemoglobin levels. This makes it appear as though an athlete has an iron deficiency. However, sports anemia is not "true" anemia, and it does not impair the oxygen-carrying capacity of hemoglobin. With continued training, sports anemia disappears on its own.

Iron has recently received attention in the media because of research that links high iron intake and heart disease. Such reports, however, should not stop people from consuming adequate levels of iron. While too much iron may be harmful, too little can negatively affect health and limit athletic performance.

Good dietary sources of iron include meat, poultry, fish, eggs, vegetables, and fortified cereals. Meat sources contain a form of iron known as *heme iron*, which is more readily absorbed by the body than the non-heme iron contained in vegetables. In addition, vitamin C has been shown to enhance iron absorption. Also be aware that beverages such as coffee and tea, as well as the minerals calcium and phosphorus, can hinder iron absorption.

To make sure that you're including enough iron in your diet, take a general inventory of the foods you eat and start checking ingredient lists. It's a good idea to check with your physician before you supplement with iron so that he or she can make sure that supplementation is absolutely necessary. In addition to getting a standard test for iron, ask for a test of your *ferritin* levels. Ferritin is the storage form of iron. A ferritin test will enable your doctor to tell if your iron stores are adequate.

The PDI of iron is 10 to 20 milligrams.

Special Considerations for Women. Women athletes are especially prone to iron deficiency and anemia for two reasons. First, women lose iron due to blood loss during menstruation. This may cause iron deficiency even without the additional iron losses caused by exercise. Second, studies show that women athletes tend to have low iron intakes. Women on self-imposed calorie-restricted diets, in particular, are at a higher risk for iron deficiency.

Women who suspect that they are iron-deficient are advised to consult a physician for testing before beginning a supplemental regimen. This will pinpoint the cause of iron deficiency and determine the best course of action to correct the problem.

MANGANESE

Manganese is a trace mineral that has many important functions for athletes. It is used in energy production, protein and fat metabolism, and bone and connective-tissue formation. The body's natural antioxidant, *superoxide dismutase* (SOD), is also partly composed of manganese. All of these functions are essential for peak performance.

The richest sources of manganese are avocados, Brussels sprouts, nuts and seeds, seaweed, spinach, turnip greens, wheat germ, and whole grains.

The PDI of magnesium is 15 to 45 milligrams.

MOLYBDENUM

Although it is found only in minute quantities in the body, molybdenum is an essential mineral for the maintenance of good health. Molybdenum is a component of several important enzymes that are involved in energy production and nitrogen metabolism.

Dietary sources of molybdenum include milk, beans, cereal grains, legumes, peas, and dark green leafy vegetables.

The PDI of molybdenum is 100 to 300 micrograms.

SELENIUM

Selenium is a vital component of the antioxidant enzyme glutathione. The antioxidant activity of selenium is extremely important for athletes because it helps to protect tissues against the oxidative stress of exercise. By minimizing free-radical damage, selenium, in combination with other major antioxidants, can help to reduce recovery time.

As with iodine, the selenium content of a food is dependent upon the selenium content of the soil in which the food is grown. Selenium can be found in varying contents in Brazil nuts, meat, seafood, kidney, liver, and whole grains.

The PDI of selenium is 100 to 300 micrograms.

ZINC

Although it occurs in a very small quantity in the body, zinc plays a role in many metabolic functions. It is part of more than a hundred enzymes that help metabolize carbohydrate, fat, and protein for energy, minimize free-radical damage, and synthesize DNA. Some of these enzymes are also factors in growth and cell replication. Zinc also enhances the actions of vitamin D, which is vital in calcium absorption. And, because it aids in the growth and repair of muscle tissues, zinc is especially important to help athletes recover from the rigors of training.

Meat, whole-grain products, liver, eggs, seafood, herring, oysters, oatmeal, and maple syrup are all known to be food sources rich in zinc.

The PDI of zinc is 15 to 60 milligrams.

CONCLUSION

There's growing evidence that many of us are suffering from some form of micronutrient deficiency. In general, our diets do not provide the nourishment that our bodies require for optimum health. The fact is, the nutritional guidelines that we have followed for more than fifty years provide us only with the recommended minimum amounts of vitamins and minerals needed for survival. It's rapidly becoming clear, however, that we should not just eat to survive—we need to take in adequate quantities of vitamins and minerals to help our bodies function at their best.

Obviously, athletes must focus on maintaining optimum health because an athlete's level of health ultimately determines his or her level of performance. However, physically active people often need more of the essential micronutrients, such as calcium, iron, and the electrolytes, to compensate for the amount they lose during exercise. At the same time, training requires a high output of energy, which only the increased consumption of nutrients can provide. Fortunately, as you learned, recent innovations in sports nutrition have resulted in a new set of standards, called the Performance Daily Intakes, to help athletes meet their increased nutritional needs for maximum performance. The PDIs not only provide guidance to help athletes meet their requirements for the hustle and bustle of everyday life, they also ensure maximum nutritional support for the rigors of training and competition.

Enhancing Performance, Reducing Injuries, and Improving Recovery with Sports Supplements

Have you ever bought and tried a sports-nutrition supplement that didn't live up to its claims? Or have you found that when confronted with an overabundance of sports-nutrition products, you simply couldn't decide which would offer the greatest benefits? You're not alone. Faced with manufacturers' competing claims, other athletes also have trouble selecting supplements that will effectively enhance performance.

Because so many of the products available today base their claims on hype rather than on sound scientific knowledge, it's often very difficult to determine if they can really improve muscle performance—or if they may do more harm than good. To aid you in your quest to select practical, research-proven products, this chapter reviews some of the more popular supplements that are effective at delaying muscular fatigue, preventing joint distress, and aiding in muscle and joint recovery.

CAFFEINE

Caffeine is a naturally occurring compound that is found in coffee, tea, chocolate, cola, and several herbs. Many people use it in food, drink, and/or pill form as a stimulant or to increase alertness. A good percentage of the population relies on a caffeinated drink to function every morning or for a boost during the day.

For athletes, however, caffeine is more than just a means to wake up in the morning. Studies have shown that caffeine can also benefit performance. When you exercise, your muscles always use some combination of carbohydrate and fat for fuel. Caffeine increases your body's use of fatty acids for energy, which in turn helps to spare glycogen. It also acts as a nervous-system stimulant to provide a mental boost that helps athletes through strenuous training sessions or long events.

This is all well and good—until we are reminded of caffeine's negative effects on health and, consequently, on performance. When you take caffeine in excess—in any form—it can irritate your stomach lining and disrupt sleep. In addition, it acts as a diuretic, which can accelerate dehydration. These are all side effects that you can do without, both in your day-to-day life and during exercise.

If you habitually drink caffeinated coffee or soda, you need to know that you have probably built up a tolerance to caffeine, meaning that you will require greater amounts to see any improvement in performance. To make matters worse, if you are accustomed to daily large amounts of coffee or caffeinated beverages and you try to cut back, you will most likely have to endure withdrawal symptoms before your body can overcome its dependency. Therefore, it's best to use caffeine sparingly, and only periodically, to enhance workouts.

Recommended Dosage

If you do decide to use caffeine to enhance performance during extended exercise, you'll find that 2 milligrams per pound of your body weight taken about thirty to sixty minutes before activity may be your optimal dose. For a 160-pound athlete, this means about 320 milligrams before exercise to provide an *ergogenic* (performance-enhancing) effect. This amount can be obtained from about four 5-ounce cups of brewed (drip method) coffee, each containing 80 milligrams of caffeine. A 5-ounce cup of brewed tea provides 40 milligrams of caffeine, or about half the caffeine of 5 ounces of coffee. Remember that you want to refrain from drinking carbonated beverages such as soft drinks during long-term exercise because they can cause gastrointestinal distress. Gas can make you feel full, so that you will not drink as much during and after exercise to rehydrate. If you really want to drink a refreshing caffeine-containing soda before or during exercise, open the bottle for several hours before use to help "defuse" the carbonation.

There are also more and more sports gels and bars that are appearing on the market that contain caffeine as part of their ingredients. You may want to experiment with these during training and see if they help your performance.

Do keep in mind, however, that at these levels, caffeine may induce the secretion of stomach acid, which can lead to heartburn. In addition, caffeine's diuretic effect will cause increased water loss through urine in the thirty minutes to two hours after ingestion. This may compound the amount of water that's sweated out during exercise, greatly increasing your chances of becoming dangerously dehydrated. As with all things related to nutrition, each individual should evaluate caffeine's effects upon his or her body and consume it at levels that take advantage of its beneficial effects but minimize the adverse effects of excess intake.

Some scientists have stated that the difference between taking caffeine (coffee, cola, Vivarin, No-Doz) and amphetamines in competition is a matter of ethics. A similar matter of ethics could be questioned in the use of carbohydrate loading or excessive vitamin supplements. These also can be considered forms of doping. To complicate matters, the International Olympic Committee has been flip-flopping on the issue of caffeine over the years. At one time it was illegal, then for a period of time it was legal, and then levels of more than 15 micrograms (mcg) of caffeine per milliliter of urine became grounds for disqualification. Now, the level has been changed again, and an amount greater than 12 micrograms per milliliter is considered doping. As an example, to reach this limit, one would have to consume approximately six to eight cups of coffee in one sitting and be tested within two to three hours. However, there are other sources of caffeine, such as colas, aspirin, and Vivarin that may cause excessive levels in the urine. During the course of a day's competition, an athlete may inadvertently take in too much caffeine and show up positive on testing.

Caffeine is a legal nutritional supplement, and athletes are free to experiment with it. But caution must be exercised. While it will most likely increase endurance performance, its improper use could have detrimental side effects. Lastly, caffeine's improper use could lead to disqualification in competition.

Nutritional Ergogenic Aids

As long as competitive sports have existed, athletes have attempted to improve their performance by ingesting a variety of nutritional supplements. At one time, it was believed that eating certain foods would impart the desirable characteristics of the food source on the person who ate them. For example, some athletes would eat the meat of a bull before competition in an effort to increase strength and courage. From elixirs in ancient Greece to modern-day carbohydrate beverages, athletes have used different substances to improve performance or reverse their body's fatigue.

The term *ergogenic aid* is defined as a work- or performance-enhancing aid. Any substance, technique, or piece of equipment used in an effort to improve performance may be considered an ergo-

continued

genic aid. The most often used and abused ergogenic aids, however, are nutritional ergogenic aids. Pick up any health-and-fitness magazine and you can hardly turn a page without seeing an advertisement for a new product or compound being hyped to improve performance.

Advertisers prey on athletes, who have a burning desire to improve performance, by making claims like the following:

- Some substances such as supplements derived from plant sterols (cholesterol and its derivatives, including steroid hormones and various vitamins) provide as much as 50 percent of the biological activity of anabolic steroids.
- The mineral boron promotes testosterone synthesis in the body.
- Royal jelly (produced by worker bees and fed to the queen bee) benefits endurance performance.
- Carnitine helps you lose weight.

In each case, there is virtually no scientific research to support the claims of these products. The National Council Against Health Fraud's Ergogenic Aids Task Force has published guidelines called "Deceptive Tactics Used in Marketing Purported Ergogenic Aids" in the *National Strength and Conditioning Association Journal*. They reviewed claims made by forty-five companies that sell ergogenic aids and outlined practices that they believe to be unacceptable. Here are the nine points that were highlighted in that article:

- **Misrepresentation of research.** Research is taken out of context, or unmerited conclusions are referred to it. "University tested" may mean only that someone inside a univer-

continued

sity was involved, with no evidence of whether the study had merit. Endorsement by a team may mean that the company sent the team samples and they were not sent back.

- **False statements.** "We are currently doing double-blind research" is a common statement, but it is rarely true.
- **No right to documentation of claim.** "Research not for public review" thwarts the consumer's right to documentation of performance claims.
- **Testimonials.** A person may claim that a substance was effective for him or her, but even a placebo, or dummy pill, will produce results in some people that will make them believe a substance is effective.
- **Patents.** A patent says nothing about the effectiveness of a product.
- **Inappropriately used research.** Research that is poorly controlled, outdated, taken out of context, not peer-reviewed, or from Eastern European sources cannot be relied upon.
- **Publicity and articles.** These are planted in publications to avoid possible prosecution for the same false and misleading claims if made in an ad.
- **Mail-order evaluations.** Computerized evaluations conveniently find that the consumer needs the products the company wants to sell.
- **Anabolic measurements based on nitrogen balance.** These measurements don't correlate to increased lean body mass and therefore do not prove the worth of very high-protein supplements.

It's okay to be a skeptic. In fact, it's your responsibility. Question claims, especially ones that seem too good to be true. Re-

continued

member, just because something appears in print does not mean that it's true.

Below are several questions to ask when purchasing a nutritional supplement or when evaluating the manufacturer's advertising or literature:

- What scientific evidence is available to support the claim?
- Where were the scientific studies conducted?
- By whom were the studies conducted? What were the researchers' and laboratories' qualifications?
- Do the researchers have a commercial or financial interest in the company?
- Where was the study published? Was it published in a reputable scientific journal or in a popular magazine?
- Was the study peer-reviewed?
- Are there any other studies to support or deny the claims?
- What do recognized experts in the field say about the research?
- Who are the experts? What are their credentials?

As long as athletes and other active individuals strive for improved performance, quicker recovery, and increased muscle mass, new nutritional supplements and products will be available to help aid in their success. Evaluation of these products by the nutritional-supplement industry, athletes, coaches, consumer and trade publications, and the general media will remain an ongoing process. And it will require you to ask the right questions. In the end, good science and the truth is the antidote to imprecise research and claims.

CREATINE

Remember creatine's role in energy production? As we discussed in Chapter 2, our bodies use phosphate from creatine phosphate (CP) to quickly replenish ATP from ADP. The more energy the muscles store, the better they can perform in events that require explosive power, such as weightlifting, sprinting, jumping, football, hockey, and soccer, to name a few. By consuming creatine, your body can, in effect, make more CP, which will aid in the regeneration of more ATP, enabling your muscles to work at a higher intensity. The body can manufacture creatine; it is also present in food and is available in supplemental form.

It's important to note that, so far, only one study has investigated the influence of creatine supplementation on performance in exercise that lasts five to thirty minutes, and there have been no conclusive studies concerning creatine's benefits for exercise lasting more than thirty minutes. Dr. Paul Balsom from Sweden showed that performance time during a six-kilometer trail run greater than twenty minutes in duration was actually impaired after creatine supplementation. This longer running time may have been a result of increased body weight due to a creatine-induced increase in muscle mass, or it may have been simply a reflection of the highly aerobic nature of the exercise task.

The benefits of creatine supplementation for endurance athletes have been heavily researched, especially in the last few years, and have proven that creatine can, in fact, extend endurance. In one study, subjects who were given 20 grams of creatine a day for five days were able to exercise for a significantly longer duration than those who were given a placebo.

Another study showed that creatine supplementation can cause a significant increase in lactate threshold (the point at which lactic acid begins to accumulate in the body), from 67 to 74 percent. This study was conducted with nineteen male and nine female trained runners who ingested 20 grams of creatine a day for seven to eight days. No significant differences were observed in maximal work capacity, however.

One study, completed by Dr. Louise Burke of the Australian Sports Institute, did not show any improvement in swimmers who supplemented with creatine in events such as 25-, 50- and 100-meter sprints. Again, this is likely due to an increase in weight resulting from increased muscle mass. Athletes, such as swimmers, who can be slowed down by weight gain will probably want to avoid supplementing with creatine. Individuals who supplement with creatine monohydrate can expect to increase their weight while decreasing their percentage of body fat, when supplementation is combined with physical training. Endurance athletes are strongly cautioned to avoid putting on too much muscle mass as a result of creatine supplementation because the energy cost of carrying excessive body weight during exercise is increased.

Recommended Dosage

The form of creatine used in all studies in which creatine shows an ergogenic (performance-enhancing) effect is *creatine monohydrate.* Several quality creatine products are available in capsule and powder form. A single 5-gram serving of powder is approximately 1 teaspoon. This should be dissolved in some form of liquid immediately before consumption.

The best method for increasing and maintaining elevated creatine stores is to start with a five-day loading phase, followed by a maintenance period. During the loading phase, a total of 20 to 25 grams of creatine should be taken in 5-gram doses, every two to three hours throughout the day. If you experience any problems, including gastrointestinal problems, when consuming large doses of creatine, you may consider taking 3 grams a day for thirty days during the loading phase.

Since more stored creatine will, together with ATP, produce more energy, it is particularly important to optimize creatine uptake into muscle tissue during this phase. One way to achieve this is to supplement with carbohydrate, which can increase creatine uptake into muscle and reduce excretion of creatine in the urine. Thus, during the loading phase, carbohydrate should be consumed with the creatine. Once the five-day loading period is complete, the muscles should be fully saturated, which makes further increases unlikely. At this point, maintaining levels of creatine in the muscles becomes an important factor.

A much lower intake of creatine is required to maintain elevated creatine stores. As little as 2 grams a day of creatine will maintain elevated creatine stores in individuals who do not exercise. However, during training, athletes will use more creatine from their stores to resynthesize ATP for energy. In this case, a more appropriate dosage is about 3 to 5 grams a day. In addition, athletes who weigh more than 220 pounds may try taking as much as 10 grams a day, because increased muscle mass demands increased levels of creatine.

HMB

A popular anabolic supplement is *beta-hydroxy beta-methylbutyrate* (HMB). Because HMB is a breakdown product of the amino acid leucine, it aids protein synthesis in the body, which helps to maximize the muscle-building aim of exercise. Although it is found in small quantities in some foods, such as catfish and citrus fruits, athletes may want to supplement with commercial products to secure the full benefits of HMB.

In a study published by S. Nissen and colleagues from the University of Iowa, forty-one male volunteers ranging in age from nineteen to twenty-nine, each weighing an average of 180 pounds, were randomly assigned one of two HMB dosages or a placebo. The results showed that subjects gained lean body mass according to the dosage that they had been administered. Total strength for upper- and lower-body exercises increased by an average of 8 percent in subjects who did not supplement. This is compared with a 13 percent average increase in the males who took 1.5 grams of HMB, and an 18.4 percent average increase in subjects who were administered 3-gram dosages. Researchers also found that subjects who supplemented with HMB were able to lift more weight than subjects who did not supplement during all three weeks. The results of this study clearly indicate that HMB supplementation can improve muscle strength and lean body mass.

The benefits that were apparent with HMB supplementation occurred independently of the level of protein that test subjects consumed. However, it's important to note that even the subjects consuming the lesser amount of protein were still ingesting large amounts. Therefore, it's possible that a protein intake considered normal by non-bodybuilding standards would limit the benefits of HMB.

Recently, a study conducted by researchers at Iowa State University showed that HMB can also benefit endurance runners. These runners took either HMB or a placebo, in pill form, every day for five weeks. After the fifth week of supplementation, the test subjects ran a twenty-kilometer race to test for muscle damage and soreness after exercise. After the race, runners were tested for evidence of muscle damage and loss of strength. The extent of muscle damage was determined by measuring blood levels of creatine kinase (CK), which, as you may remember, increases with an increase in muscle damage. The HMB group had significantly lower levels of CK, meaning that there was less evidence of muscle damage when compared with the placebo group. Measurements of post-race leg strength showed that the HMB group lost less muscle strength as well. This study has been the first of its kind to highlight HMB's potential in runners to reduce muscle damage and help maintain muscle strength. All of the available research thus far has shown HMB to be very beneficial as a muscle builder and protector.

Recommended Dosage

Researchers now recommend supplementation with 3 to 5 grams of HMB per day to build muscle and increase muscle strength. All of the studies to date have shown that HMB is safe and effective for both men and women. Human studies have been conducted with up to 4 grams of HMB administered daily for up to four weeks. The researchers report no toxicity at these levels.

PHOSPHATIDYLSERINE

Phosphatidylserine (PS), one of the body's phospholipids, is an integral part of the structure and maintenance of cell membranes. Recently, attention has turned to PS as a sports supplement because it can actually help to counteract some of the negative effects of strenuous training. In particular, PS has been shown to reduce the levels of the stress hormone cortisol, which accelerates protein breakdown for energy.

The results of at least three clinical trials have suggested that phosphatidylserine limits exercise-induced increases in cortisol. In the first study, investigators found that a 75-milligram dose of PS, when administered intravenously, reduced cortisol release by about 33 percent. Similar results were evident when the study was repeated with 800 milligrams of PS administered in an oral dose. Based on these studies, PS can soften the severity of the body's response to exercise stress.

A study by Thomas Fahey, Ed.D., of California State University in Chico, confirmed these results. Eleven college students who trained with weights were given 800 milligrams of oral PS daily and then put through a vigorous, whole-body weight workout four times a week. This regimen was intentionally designed to overtrain the students. Cortisol levels were found to be 20 percent lower in individuals supplementing with PS. Dr. Fahey concluded that up to 800 milligrams of PS is effective in suppressing the cortisol response.

Reducing cortisol has the potential to dramatically improve the way athletes train and use supplements for recovery. Phosphatidylserine can help athletes to recover faster after strenuous workouts by reducing muscle breakdown and the accompanying muscle soreness. It's logical to conclude that PS may even enhance the effectiveness of carbohydrate/ protein recovery drinks.

Recommended Dosage

Phosphatidylserine is not available in large quantities in the diet. According to rough estimates, in fact, the total amount of PS that is taken in from food hardly reaches 80 milligrams per day. In light of the recent research, athletes may benefit from supplementation to meet the recommended dosage of 400 to 800 milligrams of PS daily.

Until recently, concentrated PS was commercially available only in a bovine-derived product. However, this product was considered to be potentially hazardous because of the threat of mad cow disease. And safe forms of PS, which were derived from vegetables, contained only trace amounts of the phospholipid. Fortunately, a new form of concentrated PS, which is derived from soybeans, has proven to be a safe and effective source for supplementation.

MSM

Methylsulfonylmethane (MSM) has been turning up in countless sport- and arthritis-related supplements in the last few years. MSM is naturally found in human blood and organs, but commercially, it is made from DMSO (dimethyl sulfoxide) that has been oxygenated to become DMSO2 (dimethyl sulfone), turning it from a liquid to a granular product. Like SAMe (S-adenosylmethionine), its sulfur content is thought to help explain its ability to aid in arthritis therapy. Sulfur concentration in the cartilage of arthritis patients is only about one-third of the normal level, and since sulfur is needed to form connective tissue, supplemental sulfur can help. MSM also has anti-inflammatory properties and helps to normalize the immune system, which is important in autoimmune conditions and rheumatoid arthritis.

One recent study found that patients with degenerative arthritis who took 2,250 milligrams of MSM daily gained more than 80 percent control of pain within six weeks of starting the study compared to those who took a placebo. A recent preliminary study with MSM found that people suffering from sprains, strains, and other athletic injuries had better recovery than people in the control group, with 40 percent fewer office visits before recovery.

The recent popularity of MSM prompted another clinical study to validate the anecdotal claims made by athletes who use the nutritional supplement to relieve sports injuries.

The results were impressive. Of the twenty-four patients involved in the study, those taking MSM had a significant level of recovery (58.3 percent) compared with those on placebo (33.3 percent). The study was conducted in the clinical practice of Drs. Daniel Sanchez and Mark Grosman. The doctors treat a large number of athletic injuries each day. Each of the patients involved in the study suffered from acute injuries sustained during athletic activity. Each was treated with similar therapy and each received unmarked capsules of either a placebo or MSM. Four of the patients taking the MSM reported the disappearance of symptoms after taking the capsules for a very short period of time.

The study reinforced the findings of previous studies, which have shown that MSM has a very low level of toxicity and has few, if any, side effects for the user. In addition to the positive health factors, the economic advantages of MSM illustrated by this study can't be ignored. The compound itself is inexpensive and easy to use. In addition, the 40 percent reduction in office visits for those on MSM versus the placebo make it an invaluable, cost-effective treatment for sports injuries.

Recommended Dosage

MSM has demonstrated the remarkable ability to reduce or eliminate muscle soreness and leg and back cramps, particularly in geriatric patients who have such cramps during the night or after long periods of inactivity, and in athletes after high physical stress.

Marathon runners and other athletes who compete or exercise vigorously can learn from trainers of million-dollar racehorses. Trainers will administer MSM to their prize horses both before a race to prevent muscle soreness and afterward to lessen the risk of cramping. In one study, delayed muscle soreness, which can last for many days after intense exercise, was gone in two to three days in people who had taken 1,000 to 3,000 milligrams of MSM per day in split dosages for the preceding six months. Common dosages are 2,000 to 4,000 milligrams a day.

GLUCOSAMINE FOR JOINT DISTRESS

Many individuals are familiar with the pain and discomfort of joint pain. In the knee, for example, excessive damage to the cartilage can occur by excessive trauma, such as continued running on hard surfaces, malposition of joints, or multiple traumatic blows to a joint over a number of years (caused, say, by repetitive hits to the knee from your days of playing high school and college football).

Cartilage is a plasticlike tissue; it is made up of thick bundles of collagen. Like a tapestry, collagen fibers are woven in many directions within the joint to form the shape and size of cartilage. As cartilage begins to merge with bone, it becomes more calcified or hardened, forming a seamless bond to bone. Cartilage in a joint such as the knee helps cushion joints every time the knee moves, as part of the body's shock-absorbing system.

In the knee, much of the pain, discomfort, inflammation, and eventual osteoarthritis occur because of damage to the cartilage that leaves the heads of the leg bones—the tibia and femur—in contact with each other, causing pain and increased inflammation.

One study of athletes looked at glucosamine, a supplement that has helped relieve the pain of inflammation of osteoarthritis. A total of sixty-eight athletes with cartilage damage in their knees were given 1,500 milligrams of glucosamine sulfate daily for forty days, and then 750 milligrams for about ninety to one hundred days. Of the sixty-eight athletes, fifty-two had complete disappearance of their symptoms and resumed full athletic training. After four to five months, athletes were able to train at pre-injury rates. While no control group was used in this study, glucosamine sulfate supplementation was associated with recovery in the majority of the athletes. A follow-up twelve months later showed no signs of cartilage damage in any of the athletes.

To understand how glucosamine works in supporting joint health, one has to look at the structure of collagen and its components. In the cartilage, *glycosaminoglycans* (GAGs) are the tissue framework that collagen holds on to. Collagen and GAGs together continuously construct and reconstruct your cartilage.

This is where glucosamine comes into play. Glucosamine is the major precursor of GAGs. But even more important, the making of glucosamine from glucose and glutamine is the body's rate-limiting step in GAG production, and hence a rate-limiting step in building and rebuilding cartilage after trauma. Following cartilage trauma or tearing, this limit does not allow the body to make sufficient GAGs for optimal healing. In addition, as one ages, the ability to convert glucose to glucosamine declines because of a reduction in the level of the converting enzyme glucosamine synthetase. This is where oral glucosamine comes in. Taking glucosamine supplements can increase GAG levels significantly.

THE HEALING POWER OF PROTEOLYTIC ENZYMES

The process of inflammation is governed by numerous enzymes, especially the body's own proteolytic enzymes. They eliminate the inflammatory debris and initiate restitution.

The process can be supported and accelerated by the use of supplemental proteolytic enzymes, such as papain, bromelain, and trypsin. They keep the pathological process from spreading and considerably reduce the duration of the disease. Proteolytic enzymes accelerate the inflammatory process necessary for the healing of an injury or wound. This acceleration means, on the one hand, that the work of damage control, repair, and new tissue generation is carried out more forcefully and precisely, and thus, completed more swiftly. On the other hand, it means there may be a temporary increase in the sensory and visual effects produced by the inflammation. Often, there is more swelling, redness, heat, and pain, which are signs that the body is working to heal the injury.

These "protease" enzyme nutrients are found in all living cells. In supplemental form, they may be one of the best sources of natural healing for sports injuries and joint problems. Two of the most common come from fruit: papain from papayas and bromelain from pineapples.

The clinical evidence supporting the use of proteases is encouraging. Football players at the University of Pittsburgh who were given proteases found that minor injuries healed faster, compared with injuries that were treated with a placebo. At the University of Delaware, athletes using protease supplements were able to cut recovery time due to injury from 8.4 to 3.9 days.

There are many varieties of proteolytic enzymes on the market, so selecting a commercial product can be difficult. Select protease products that are "enteric coated" to help resist breakdown by stomach acid. Formulations with more than one type of protease enzyme should also be used in healing. The more proteases that are listed, the greater the effect. Combinations of bromelain, papain, trypsin, and chymotrypsin are best.

Although proteases can help reduce pain in addition to speeding repair, they don't stop pain as do prescription painkillers and aspirin.

CONCLUSION

In today's sports world, it's becoming increasingly popular for athletes to use natural supplements to optimize recovery and enhance performance. By increasing the rate of energy production and replenishment, protecting against muscle damage, and maximizing muscle building, these products may be just what some athletes need to gain that extra competitive edge. However, misconceptions about the relationship between certain supplements and exercise performance can lead athletes to expect unrealistic results. Researchers are still gathering information about the benefits—and possible side effects—of many of these cutting-edge products.

In any case, it's important to keep the benefits of sports supplements in the proper perspective. These products should be incorporated into your regular training diet to enhance recovery and performance, rather than being used alone. As always, it's best to do your homework and to remain informed of the latest research on the products you choose.

Since injuries reduce training time and prevent participation in events, any reduction in healing time will greatly aid athletic endeavors. It is puzzling why nutrients with known roles in connective tissue health and healing have been barely studied and used in athletic training. The few exciting studies show such promising results. Likewise, studies on the clinical benefits of supplementation with certain nutrients, including MSM and glucosamine, in treating joint and musculoskeletal problems show very promising results.

Knowing which nutrients have an impact on connective-tissue and joint health is important in preventing and possibly reversing long-term chronic injuries. However, future studies are needed in order to be able to give more specific information and recommendations on these topics. Fertile areas of research into the effects of nutrition, antioxidants, and proteases on sports health and healing abound.

Nutrition to Delay Event Fatigue

While training and post-exercise nutrition are essential for consistent performance, what you eat—and how much of it you eat—in the days and hours before competition is just as important in delaying fatigue. One of the most popular and effective nutritional methods for delaying the fatigue brought on by low glycogen stores is to first deplete the body's glycogen stores and then consume a high-carbohydrate diet in the days prior to your event. This technique is known as *carbohydrate loading* or *glycogen supercompensation*.

During regular training, an athlete should consume a proportion of nutrients that contains approximately 60 percent of calories from carbohydrate, 25 percent from fat, and 15 percent from protein. Starting a few days before competition, however, endurance athletes who "carbo load" will boost their carbohydrate intake to up to 70 percent of dietary calories.

This chapter discusses the nutritional basis for carbohydrate loading and presents two effective methods for achieving exceptional results. In addition, while the meals in the days leading up to competition will have the greatest impact on performance, what you eat and drink in the hours before competition is also important to your performance.

CARBOHYDRATE DEPLETION AND REPLENISHMENT

During the 1970s, researchers studied the effects of diets containing various levels of carbohydrate on performance during intensive exercise. They found that when subjects exercised intensely to deplete their glycogen stores and then consumed a carbohydrate-rich diet each day for several days afterward, their endurance was significantly increased.

As you will remember from earlier chapters, your muscles use carbohydrate as their primary source of energy during intensive exercise. Whatever is not used is transported to the muscles and liver, where it is stored as glycogen for future use. When your body needs energy, glycogen stores are converted back to glucose and burned as fuel. Even though glycogen is your body's most important source of energy, your body's capacity to store glycogen is limited. When you have used most or all of the available glycogen supply, your body begins to break down fat into fatty acids for energy. In addition, during long-term exercise, some of the amino acids that make up muscle tissue are used to fuel your body's activity, which negatively affects your efforts to build up muscle tissue.

Carbohydrate loading helps to ensure that your glycogen stores will not be so quickly depleted during exercise. Carbohydrate loading also enables your muscles to store glycogen more efficiently, so that when you enter the days of high-carbohydrate consumption, your muscles become supercompensated with glycogen.

WHO BENEFITS FROM CARBOHYDRATE LOADING?

Carbohydrate loading is a useful method for helping athletes to avoid "hitting the wall," so in general, endurance athletes reap the greatest benefits from this dietary regimen. These athletes include long-distance swimmers, cross-country skiers, soccer players, long-distance runners (especially marathoners), triathletes, and long-distance cyclists. For the most part, any athlete participating in an event lasting more than ninety minutes will find carbohydrate loading to be highly effective. While it is unlikely that you will hit the wall in an event lasting fewer than ninety minutes, such as a basketball or football game or a track-and-field event, you may still find carbohydrate loading to be moderately beneficial. Just try tapering off training a few days before competition and boosting the percentage of carbohydrate in your diet.

You should be aware that some athletes should not practice carbohydrate loading at all. Athletes who need to meet weight-class requirements should avoid carbohydrate loading because of the high caloric intake during the days preceding competition. Other athletes state that they feel bloated, or that their muscles feel "heavy" after a week of a high-carbohydrate diet and reduced training, and they complain that this hinders, rather than enhances, their performance. This is because, for every gram of carbohydrate that you store, you also store between 3 and 5 grams of water. If you are considering carbohydrate loading before an important competition, you should make a trial run before a minor competition or during the off-season to see how your body responds.

There have not been any consistent reports of long-term gains in body weight with fluctuating glycogen levels. Any weight that an athlete puts on from carbohydrate loading is most likely due to water weight gain. Interestingly enough, there may actually be an advantage to gaining this water weight before competition: extra water can be used to help cool you down by allowing for sweating during high-intensity exercise in the heat.

METHODS OF CARBOHYDRATE LOADING

There are two general methods of carbohydrate loading that are considered to be effective. The first method was built upon the early research on glycogen depletion and replenishment, and includes very intense training in the days prior to competition. The second method is a modified version of the first regimen, and it has proved to be less stressful on the body but equally effective.

The Classical Regimen of Carbohydrate Loading

The classical regimen of carbohydrate loading became very popular in the 1970s. This technique requires you to complete intense training sessions for three days and maintain a low-carbohydrate diet in order to deplete your body's glycogen stores. Following the three-day depletion phase is a three-day period during which you should cut back on training intensity and consume a diet that includes 70 percent of calories from carbohydrate. The classical regimen has been shown to increase a trained athlete's muscle glycogen stores by two to two and a half times, which results in extended endurance.

This method of carbohydrate loading does have drawbacks, however. Some athletes are not comfortable training to exhaustion four or five days before competition. Many also find that training becomes difficult when glycogen stores are at such low levels because they simply have less energy. As a result, the quality of the athlete's workout suffers, leaving some competitors feeling that they are not properly prepared for their events. In addition, low glycogen stores can lead to fatigue and improper form, which increases the risk of injury.

Fat Loading for Endurance?

Recently, some individuals have advocated the practice of "fat loading" to spare glycogen stores and increase endurance. The reasoning behind this is that fat is the body's most energy-rich nutrient, containing 9 calories in 1 gram. Therefore, when compared with carbohydrate, which has only 4 calories in 1 gram, fat is shown to contain more than twice the energy.

So why haven't endurance athletes started eating cookies for breakfast or munching potato chips for a pre-exercise energy boost? The most obvious reason seems to be that, from a nutritional standpoint, a diet loaded with refined, processed foods that are high in the "wrong" kinds of fats is a health disaster waiting to happen. Pertaining to sports, high-fat diets have been shown to actually reduce glycogen stores and, as a result, to impair performance. In one study, individuals ate a diet consisting of 76 percent fat for four days. After the fourth day, when the subjects were asked to run until exhaustion, those who had fat loaded reached exhaustion 40 percent sooner than those who had consumed a diet lower in fat.

The reason for this is that the body can't oxidize fat as well as it can glycogen during intense exercise. During exercise, only about 30 percent of your body's energy is derived from fat. And even though fat may produce more energy per gram, your body needs about 75 percent more oxygen to "burn" the fat. This puts greater stress on your cardiorespiratory system.

When all's said and done, exhaustion during exercise is still directly linked to glycogen depletion. Therefore, to forestall exercise-induced fatigue, you should eat a high-carbohydrate diet during training. If you train at high intensity, you should include about

continued

3 to 5 grams of carbohydrate in your diet per pound of your body weight. If you have difficulty achieving this goal, you might find it beneficial to use a carbohydrate supplement before, during, and after training to load, sustain, and replenish glycogen stores. Also, be sure to use the guidelines presented in this chapter for carbohydrate loading prior to any competition lasting longer than ninety minutes.

The Modified Regimen of Carbohydrate Loading

Dr. Michael Sherman of Ohio State University has shown that glycogen supercompensation can be achieved through a modified regimen of carbohydrate loading. This method has been shown to raise glycogen levels comparably to the levels induced by the classical regimen—with few side effects. Dr. Sherman recommends that, during the six days before competition, athletes consume a 50 percent carbohydrate diet for three days, followed by a 70 percent carbohydrate diet for three days. During this six-day period, exercise duration is progressively decreased: from ninety minutes on the first day, to about forty minutes on the second and third days, to approximately twenty minutes on the fourth and fifth days, to very light exercise or total rest on the final day. This regimen is outlined in Table 16.1 on page 221.

But how do you know that you are obtaining the proper percentage of carbohydrate from your diet? One way is to go by percentage of total caloric intake. You can also consume 2 grams of carbohydrate for every pound of your body weight per day during the 50 percent days, and up to 5 grams of carbohydrate for every pound of body weight per day during the 70 percent days.

Table 16.1. Modified Regimen for Carbohydrate Loading

DAY	EXERCISE DURATION	PERCENT OF CALORIES FROM CARBOHYDRATE
1	90 minutes	50 percent
2	40 minutes	50 percent
3	40 minutes	50 percent
4	20 minutes	70 percent
5	20 minutes	70 percent
6	Rest	70 percent
7	Race	70 percent

New Spin on Carbohydrate Loading

In the newest study to tackle this problem of carbohydrate loading, Dr. Timothy Fairchild and coworkers from the University of Western Australia evaluated whether one day of high carbohydrate intake after a short bout of high-intensity exercise would result in above-normal levels of muscle glycogen.

Seven endurance-trained cyclists participated in the study. The subjects' normal diets provided an average of 3.3 grams of carbohydrate per pound of lean body mass, which slightly tapered leading up to the testing day. After a five-minute warmup, the fasted cyclists rode for 150 seconds at 130% of maximum oxygen consumption and then sprinted for 30 seconds.

For the next twenty-four hours, the subjects consumed 5.1 grams per pound of body weight of high-carbohydrate foods with a high glycemic index. The subjects started consuming carbohydrate within twenty minutes of terminating exercise, kept a diet and physical-activity record, and did not engage in any physical training. Carbohydrate-rich beverages provided more than 80% of carbohydrate intake to ensure compliance with the carbohydrate-loading diet.

This novel carbohydrate-loading regimen significantly increased muscle-glycogen stores by 82% from the pre-sprint ride levels. This is the first research study to build large muscle-glycogen stores in as little time as twenty-four hours through carbohydrate loading and high-intensity exercise.

This carbohydrate-loading protocol is faster than other regimens while still providing comparable muscle-glycogen levels. The primary advantage of this rapid regimen is that the diet and exercise strategies required to carbohydrate-load can be initiated twenty-four hours before competition with minimal disruption to training and event preparation. Perhaps more significantly, this method proved equal to or better than any of the more traditional carbo-loading methods that have been studied.

So, after your final pre-race run or ride, which should include about three minutes of super-maximal exercise, concentrate on high-carbohydrate, quickly digestible foods and drinks for the twenty-four hours before your race. Good sources are whole-grain breads and rolls, rice, potatoes, pasta, and, of course, a high-carbohydrate/protein drink.

BOOSTING YOUR CARBOHYDRATE INTAKE

If you've ever tried to maintain a diet that includes a large percentage of calories from carbohydrate, you know that it's no easy task! Remember that gram for gram, carbohydrate contains less than half the calories of fat. You may want to use high-carbohydrate drinks to supplement your carbohydrate intake. These will allow you to consume large amounts of carbohydrates without the added bulk.

Whichever regimen you choose to follow, keep in mind that all kinds of carbohydrate can help replenish glycogen stores. However, before a training session, those with low glycemic indexes work best because they release glucose into the bloodstream slowly, allowing for a steady release of carbohydrate into your bloodstream. (For a discussion of glycemic indexes, see the inset "Glycemic Index" on page 96.)

In addition, try to increase your portions of complex carbohydrates. Foods such as cereals, pasta, whole-wheat breads, grains, and beans will provide you with vitamins, minerals, fiber, and protein, as well as carbohydrate. Try to stay away from simple sugars, since they tend to be low in vitamins, minerals, and fiber. The rest of your diet should contain foods that are good sources of protein and fat.

PRE-EXERCISE AND PRE-EVENT MEALS

The timing of your last meal before competition or hard training will depend on the intensity and duration of the competition. Begin by experimenting with the timing of your meals. You want to enter most events with an empty stomach at the time of competition, yet you don't want to feel hungry or weak on the line or starting block. For many people, this means eating their last meal two to four hours before the event.

Additional factors that affect eating and exercise timing are fitness level, exercise intensity, and stress. A highly fit individual can perform more intense exercise after eating without placing a great burden on the digestive system. Mild exercise, such as easy cycling and walking, after eating can be tolerated by many athletes. For example, in the Tour de France, many athletes can be seen eating on the starting line, since they know the first few hours of the race will be at a moderate pace and they may be racing for up to seven hours. Being nervous about competition will also affect how much and how far before competition you decide to eat.

Pre-exercise meals are important; however, it is your nutritional habits during the previous days that have the greatest impact on performance. A great deal of controversy exists over the composition and timing of pre-event meals. Most research indicates that consuming a pre-event meal with a low glycemic index (GI) is beneficial. Low GI foods should provide for a slow release of glucose into the circulation without causing a surge in insulin. By providing a steady source of carbohydrate to exercising muscles when glycogen levels are low, fatigue may be delayed. Low GI foods consumed before exercise may provide enhanced fuel substrates for active muscles during the later stages of exercise and replenishment of glycogen during the post-exercise period. The meal should contain approximately 300 to 600 calories primarily from carbohydrate with small amounts of protein and fat. Additionally, 2.5 milliliters of water per pound of body mass (approximately 2 cups for a 160-pound athlete) should be consumed during the hour prior to exercise to maintain hydration. The ideal timing of this pre-event meal has not been determined and should be based on individual preference. Surprisingly, most athletes can tolerate foods consumed very close to exercise without experiencing abnormal blood glucose and insulin responses. Do not eat foods prior to an event that you have not tried before.

If you are one to have a nervous stomach before competition, you may also want to experiment with liquid food supplements. These products are available in various flavors, and once again it would be wise to experiment before a training session with these products before using them in competition.

Following are two examples of quick and easy-to-prepare pre-exercise meals.

MENU ONE
1 granola bar
1 cup plain or artificially sweetened yogurt
1 cup unsweetened fruit juice or sports drink

MENU TWO
1 cup of oatmeal
1 cup of skim milk
8 ounces of a sports drink
1 piece of fruit

CONCLUSION

Haphazard eating habits in the days before competition can sabotage any athlete's performance. At some point, almost all athletes encounter obstacles during competition that they cannot overcome, such as decreased endurance, difficulty concentrating, and reduced strength. In most cases, these are problems that could have been prevented or minimized with proper pre-competition nutrition.

Competition places special demands on your body above and beyond those of training, and you must be physically prepared to meet those demands. The starting points are sound nutritional knowledge and practice. Carbohydrate loading is a valuable means to forestall fatigue and perform at peak capacity during long events. But keep in mind that carbohydrate loading is not a daily nutritional regimen for performance, and as such, it should be practiced only when necessary about a week before competition. When your event is not close at hand, you should rely on carefully balanced nutrition for overall health and optimal recovery.

Sleep and Recovery

There is mounting evidence that athletes and active individuals need plenty of sleep. Fatigue tends to accumulate quickly if you don't sleep enough, leaving you listless, unenthusiastic, and susceptible to colds. Sometimes, job and family responsibilities, late-night television, and a daily training regimen make it hard to find time for enough sleep.

But research shows that sleep has an enormous impact on the quality of life. It provides important physiological and psychological benefits integral to being competent and productive. Sleep deprivation diminishes intelligence, compromises the immune system, reduces cardiovascular performance, and may contribute to heart disease or even early death.

The reality is that the amount of sleep we need appears to be genetically determined, with the average total nighttime requirement being seven to nine hours. There are, however, healthy adults who require ten hours and others who need only four. Whatever your requirement is, if you don't meet it, you will pay a price. The initial effect of sleep deprivation is sleepiness, but in the long term, its consequences can include an interference with the release of growth hormone and a decrease in circulating levels of androgen, a muscle-building hormone. Both growth hormone and androgen are essential for muscle building, bone growth, and fat burning. Also, people who sleep seven to eight hours a night have been shown to have longer life expectancy than those who sleep either much more or much less. A twelve-year study published in the *American Journal of Cardiology* reported that men who were frequently exhausted were more than twice as likely to die from cardiovascular disease than those who did not report frequent exhaustion.

STAGES OF SLEEP

Sleep can be defined as altered states of consciousness measured by brain activity. There are five distinct states of consciousness associated with sleep: stages 1, 2, 3, and 4, and rapid eye movement (REM). The first four stages are often grouped together and referred to as nonrapid eye movement (NREM). The fifth stage is REM sleep, also called active sleep.

The following brief journey through the stages of sleep will help clarify the duration and physiological aspects of each stage:

Stage 1: This initial stage of sleep or drowsiness may last from ten seconds to ten minutes. Muscle relaxation occurs rapidly and respiration becomes shallow.

Stage 2: This is a period of light sleep and usually lasts from ten to twenty minutes. Heart rate slows and body temperature decreases. At this point, the body prepares to enter deep sleep.

Stages 3 and 4: These are the deep-sleep stages, with stage 4 being more intense than stage 3. These stages are known as slow-wave sleep.

REM Sleep: REM (rapid eye movement) sleep is the part of sleep when dreams become active. Brain activity is actually high during this stage and heart rate increases. Intense dreaming occurs during REM sleep as a result of heightened cerebral activity, but paralysis occurs simultaneously in the major voluntary muscle groups. The first period of REM sleep typically lasts ten minutes, with each recurring REM stage length-ening, and the final one lasting an hour.

Stages 1 to 4 usually last from ninety minutes to two hours, each stage lasting from ten to twenty minutes. Surprisingly, however, stages 2 and 3 repeat backward before REM sleep is achieved. So, a normal sleep cycle has an unusual and noncohesive pattern: Stage 1, 2, 3, 4, 3, 2, REM. Usu-ally, REM sleep occurs about ninety minutes after falling asleep. The five stages of sleep, including their repetition, occur cyclically. A person may complete five to six cycles in a typical night of sleep.

STAGES 3 AND 4: IMPORTANT FOR RECOVERY

Although the body is continually in a process of revitalization while sleeping, this process peaks during stages 3 and 4. Two physiological events occur during these stages that cause this effect. First, metabolic ac-tivity is at its lowest point, and second, the endocrine system increases the secretion of growth hormone. During sleep, our bodies stop all but the most essential functions so that repair and growth can be maximized. One example of this accelerated growth is demonstrated in skin tissue, which multiplies twice its normal rate during stages 3 and 4 sleep.

Hormonal responses during sleep are different in active individuals than in sedentary individuals. For example, in trained individuals, growth hormone release is lower during the first half of sleep and higher in the second half, whereas it's the opposite in nontraining individuals.

Usually, cortisol is lower in the early stages of sleep but rises consider-ably during the second half of sleep. Again, exercise can change this equa-tion. In exercising individuals, cortisol levels are higher during the first part of sleep and less later on, which makes it that much more important to sup-press cortisol early in the sleep cycle by consuming specific nutrients, such as protein, before bedtime. Testosterone levels seem to rise throughout the night. This can have dramatic implications in muscle growth and repair.

It is also important to enter the key stages 3 and 4, because if you don't, it could mean a major decline in growth hormone output, which is not optimal for total muscle recovery. Several studies have shown that growth hormone secretion is associated with stages 3 and 4 sleep and that when REM sleep declined, sleeping cortisol levels increased. One other interesting note is that cell division (*mitosis*) in many tissues, including muscle, also shows a daily surge late at night and in the early hours of the morning, often coinciding with stages 3 and 4 sleep and the rise in growth hormone, again suggesting that sleep promotes general growth and repair.

Another pitfall of sleep deprivation is its negative impact on the immune system. Significant negative effects on immune-system function can be seen after several days of partial sleep deprivation and after only a few days of total sleep deprivation. Key antioxidants and immune-system boosters, such as vitamins C and E, are important to take before bedtime, especially if you don't sleep much.

NIGHTTIME NUTRITION

Recently, attention has begun to focus on which nutrients and supplements one can take before bedtime to optimize muscle building and recovery during sleep. First, you need to be hydrated before bed so all the nutrients you consume are used effectively and muscle cells can function optimally. You need to maximize growth hormone and testosterone levels while lowering cortisol levels. Next, you need to have plenty of amino acids available for protein synthesis supported by the increase in growth and testosterone. Finally, you need an array of vitamins, minerals, and antioxidants to neutralize free radicals and provide key enzyme cofactors to support proper protein synthesis and muscle building while you sleep.

Protein

Protein is a key recovery nutrient to take before retiring for the night. Since protein synthesis occurs during sleep, it is vital to provide the body with plenty of amino acids by taking a protein drink before sleep. Many research studies show that consuming amino acids, especially essential amino acids, can stimulate protein synthesis and muscle anabolism.

The key is a combination of protein that is released slowly through metabolism while sleeping. This means a mixture of whey protein, casein, and even milk protein. Whey protein is a faster released protein and is important because it contains a high percentage of BCAAs and essential amino acids. BCAAs can increase the net protein turnover during sleep and lead to greater gains in lean muscle mass and better exercise recovery. Quality whey protein also provides key factors that can boost immune function.

Casein is a more slowly released protein, providing amino acids to the body over a longer period of the night. It has a naturally high amount of the amino acid glutamine. As discussed in earlier chapters, glutamine is essential for increasing the rate of protein synthesis while reducing breakdown in muscle tissue, along with a whole host of other great functions.

Taking 20 to 35 grams (depending on body weight) of a whey and casein blend mixed with water about one hour before going to sleep can do wonders for protein synthesis during sleep.

ZMA

ZMA, sold as a stand-alone supplement, is a special combination of zinc, magnesium and vitamin B_6 that has been found to impact athletic performance and boost testosterone levels naturally. Research has found that nightly supplementation of ZMA increased total and free testosterone levels by more than 30 percent while also increasing strength and power. Two studies have been conducted on this supplement combination, but much more research is needed on this vitamin/mineral combination in recovery nutrition.

Alpha GPC

Alpha GPC (L-alpha-glycerylphosphorylcholine) is an acetylcholine precursor derived from soy. This is a new supplement that has been shown in preliminary research to boost growth hormone levels and increase neurological function during sleep. One plus for this supplement is that small amounts (150 milligrams to 400 milligrams) seem to boost growth-hormone levels.

Vitamins, Minerals, and Antioxidants

Vitamins, minerals, and antioxidants are the key nutrients that help regulate many reactions in the body. It is known that individuals who exercise hard have a higher requirement for vitamins and minerals. Taken at night, they act as a safety net and can help maximize the process of protein synthesis and muscle repair while you sleep. In fact, one study showed that thiamine (vitamin B_1) supplementation accelerated recovery from workouts and reduced fatigue. If you are experiencing excessive muscle soreness, taking a good multivitamin/mineral formula before bed can really make a difference in recovery. Antioxidants are important because they can boost immune function and scavenge free radicals. These nutrients can be taken along with your other supplements with about 4 to 6 ounces of water or as part of your protein drink.

KEEP A REGULAR SLEEP SCHEDULE

All living people have a circadian or daily rhythm. This internal clock determines, among other things, when one feels sleepy or alert. The circadian rhythm needs consistency to perform efficiently. The importance of a consistent sleep pattern can be observed in individuals who do not have regular sleep schedules—specifically shift workers. Dr. Martin Moore-Ede, sleep specialist at the University of Harvard Medical School, says that changing one's schedule for more than two days or sleeping more than one hour longer on weekends disrupts the biological clock. Some experts believe that the primary reason people who sleep longer on the weekends report feelings of increased lethargy on Mondays is that their internal clocks have been disrupted.

Inconsistent sleep patterns not only disrupt one's internal biological clock but also tend to increase the amount of time it takes to fall asleep. Many athletes report difficulty falling asleep prior to competition, particularly the night before. The primary reason for this increased sleep latency is pre-event anxiety. Athletes who have conditioned their bodies to a particular bedtime will naturally feel drowsy and experience less difficulty going to sleep than athletes who have erratic sleep schedules.

Make Sleep a Priority

Most sleep experts recommend that adults get about eight hours of sleep if they want to wake up the next morning feeling refreshed, invigorated, and ready for a new day. The National Sleep Foundation reports, however, that most Americans get just under seven hours of sleep per night during the week, and around seven and a half hours on weekend nights.

The study claims that 35 percent of respondents report one or more symptoms of insomnia every night or almost every night, while only 21 percent rarely or never have trouble sleeping. Among the many symptoms that plague those with insomnia are:

- "Woke up feeling unrefreshed!" (40 percent)
- "Awake a lot during the night." (36 percent)
- "Difficulty falling asleep." (25 percent)
- "Woke up too early and could not get back to sleep." (24 percent)

Sleep deprivation takes its toll in a variety of ways. Those who suffer from insomnia or who don't make adequate sleep a priority

continued

may exhibit a high level of irritability in addition to feeling chronically tired, and their work performance may suffer noticeably. In addition, people with chronic illnesses are more prone to have insomnia, which significantly worsens their quality of life.

The message here is clear: Make sleep a priority.

CREATE AN OPTIMAL
SLEEPING ENVIRONMENT

Four factors typify a high-quality sleeping environment: quiet, dark, cool, and comfortable. While humans can adapt to frequent and high levels of noise during sleep, such as traffic, airplanes, and trains, low levels of noise are associated with improved sleep.

Darkness serves as an evolutionary signal to the brain that sleep should occur. In our electronic age, darkness may have to be assisted. Turning electronic devices such as a clock away from the bed, installing opaque window shades, stuffing towels around the doorjamb to eliminate light from the hallway, and using eyeshades may also be helpful in creating the darkness that signals our bodies that it is time to sleep.

Research suggests that 65°F is the optimal room temperature for sleep. Although personal preference may deviate from this norm, temperature is an important sleep variable. A room that is too hot or too cold can increase the amount of time it takes to fall asleep and the number of sleep disruptions that occur throughout the night and can decrease the overall quality of one's sleep.

While comfort of mattress, sheets, and pillow vary considerably among individuals, one generalization is fairly consistent: bigger beds are better. As a general guideline, a bed that is roughly six inches longer than your body is a good size. Sleep studies show that most humans have between forty and sixty postural shifts throughout the night. Having adequate room to freely move reduces the number of nocturnal disturbances.

THE NAP

George Sheehan, M.D., author of numerous books on running, was known to take naps to make up for lost sleep and naps to conquer fatigue and prevent exhaustion. He even took naps to make him strong and to increase his endurance.

The nap is a biological, psychological, and spiritual necessity. It renews, restores, and revives. A nap is important to the overtrained athlete who finds him- or herself more and more fatigued, whose performance is deteriorating, who lacks zest, and who is losing interest. This athlete is the one who needs more sleep at night, a nap during the day, and a break in his or her training.

Dr. Sheehan also pointed out that the nap is the answer to the self-imposed work-play week of the ordinary citizen. Few people are constructed of material strong enough to handle a program that includes a forty-hour workweek, commuting, nighttime TV, and a weekend of exhausting physical and social activities. This lifestyle leads to what must be the major deficiency disease of our age—a deficiency in rest.

When you become tired and irascible and even more difficult to live with than usual, when there is no zest in your training and your races are getting worse and worse, look around for your baby blanket and a soft spot where you can lie down. A twenty- to thirty-minute nap may do wonders to revitalize your energy and support your immune system.

SLEEP AIDS

Insomnia, difficulty falling asleep, waking repeatedly during the night, restlessness, and other sleep disturbances keep many of us from getting the rest we need—problems compounded by the fact that we are, in general, sleeping less than we used to. In addition, fatigue from a hard training session, an injury, or general muscle soreness can lead to restless sleep.

Conventional medicine relies mainly on pharmacological treatments, such as prescriptions of benzodiazepines, for serious sleep disturbances. But the drawbacks to this approach are many, including sedation hangover, impaired responses, decreased respiration, and possibly, drug dependency. Herbal sleep aids, on the other hand, can provide low-risk, widely accepted, and proven alternatives for many common sleep disorders that aren't caused by serious physical or psychological problems.

Valerian

The best-known and best-researched herbal sleep aid is valerian (*Valeriana officinalis*), which has been used for more than 500 years to help induce a good night's sleep. While the herb's restful properties have long been understood, modern consumers have only recently begun to discover ways to optimize valerian's effects. Often, people take valerian products much the same way they do conventional sleep aids—just before going to bed. Herbal treatments, however, work much differently than conventional ones.

When you take a strong prescription sedative, you feel the effects relatively quickly, usually within the hour. Herbs, generally speaking, work over a longer period of time. Clinical studies performed in the past decade indicate that valerian works best to promote natural sleep after at least two weeks of daily use. Optimum results are expected after four weeks when you take 600 milligrams two hours each night before bedtime. You can also sip a tea made from dried valerian roots, but the flavor may take some getting used to.

Generally, valerian isn't known to produce adverse side effects, although there have been some exceptions. In one study, two cases of headache were reported, in addition to one complaint of morning grogginess. In another case, a woman reported an unexpected reaction of restlessness. The good news is that no valerian dependency has been reported in all the centuries that the root has been used as a sleep aid.

Melatonin

Melatonin is a top-selling sleep-aid supplement, and it also assists with jet lag. Melatonin acts as an inner time clock in the body. It is a hormone produced by one of the most important neurotransmitters in the body, serotonin. Triggered by darkness, it is released from the pineal gland throughout the night and tells the body to sleep. Melatonin levels are sensitive to light, and as we age, the levels of it in our bodies naturally decrease.

Melatonin supplementation is most appropriate for older athletes and those who have low levels. While melatonin has not been sufficiently clinically studied for long-term use, it has been studied in low doses for short-term use. For help with sleeping and insomnia, start with doses that range from 0.5 to 3 milligrams.

Melatonin is available in liquid, tablet, and sublingual forms. Sublingual tablets dissolve under the tongue and are absorbed into the bloodstream very quickly. Time-released tablets are also available. These mimic the natural release of melatonin and have been shown to help with insomnia in a number of clinical studies. If you choose a liquid, follow the recommended drop dosage carefully, and allow it to be absorbed in the mouth. Pregnant or lactating women or people with depression or schizophrenia should not use melatonin.

THE EVENING BEFORE A RACE

Most experienced athletes begin their final preparation the night before a race. Begin by eating a high-carbohydrate dinner to top off your muscles' and liver's glycogen stores. Throughout the evening, drink plenty of fluids to reduce the chance of dehydration the next day.

Before you hit the sack, make sure all your clothing, heart-rate monitor, sunglasses, shoes, and other equipment are laid out and ready to go. You don't want to spend a sleepless night worrying whether you'll remember to pack everything.

Review your race plan. Look over the race map; imagine yourself competing on the course. Picture yourself being relaxed, and be confident of a good placing. Repeat this several times, with each session seeing yourself finishing stronger and feeling pleased about your performance.

Once you have checked everything twice, find a good book, listen to music, or turn on the television and relax. Now it is time to put the race out of your mind until race-day morning. Lastly, set two alarm clocks; this way you fall asleep knowing you'll wake up on time. Go to bed at your normal time; if you have a hard time falling asleep, try to lie there as comfortably as possible. Resting quietly is almost as restful as if you were sleeping. Remember, it's the sleep in the last few days before the race that is important, not the last few hours of sleep.

CONCLUSION

We may one day be able to set our circadian clocks as easily as we do an alarm clock. In the meantime, the solution to sleep deprivation is pretty low-tech. The first step is realizing you need more sleep. People have to recognize that sleeping is not unproductive.

Our society has created a myth that the movers and shakers of the world need less sleep than others. Thomas Edison, who probably started all this, bragged that he slept only four hours each night. How did he do it? He took at least two long naps during the day.

Nonnutritional Approaches
to Recovery

It has been said that the race is not always to the swift, but to those who keep on training. Throughout this book, we have focused on the nutritional strategies that you can use to make the most of your recovery from exercise. As the previous chapters have shown you, the R⁴ System—in combination with nutritional supplementation and natural sports products—will enable you to "keep on training" by helping you to maximize recovery and minimize muscle soreness.

Still, it would be unrealistic to believe that any nutritional program could entirely do away with muscle damage or soreness. In light of this, our guidelines for recovery would not be complete without a discussion of some nonnutritional methods that can provide relief for your hard-working muscles. For example, relaxation in a sauna or hot tub can be very therapeutic for post-exercise aches and pains. Sports massage is also an incredible recuperative tool because it helps to eliminate the physical and psychological effects of fatigue, as well as to reduce the risks of muscle injury. And simple stretching exercises during warm-up and cooldown periods are a must in keeping muscles strong and flexible and preventing damage to muscle tissue.

MASSAGE

Sports massage is not a new concept in Europe. In fact, a great number of European athletes incorporated this technique into their regular training and competition schedules long ago, and continue to appreciate its merits today. Although athletes in North America have generally been hesitant to accept massage as an integral part of training, more and more active men and women are beginning to sample the benefits for themselves.

Chris Carmichael, coach to professional cyclist Lance Armstrong, has stated, "Prior to and during major competitions, without massage and competent medical care, many athletes I've worked with would not have done as well. [Massage] relaxes the muscles, particularly after heavy training when they feel completely spent. It helps them relax and fully recover."

Researchers at the Karolinska Institute in Stockholm also found evidence to support the beneficial effects of massage. In this study, a group of competitive cyclists pedaled to exhaustion, and then had a ten-minute rest period. Half of the group received ten minutes of massage while they rested, while the other half did not receive massage. After the rest period, all of the subjects were asked to do fifty knee extensions on an exercise machine that tested leg strength. The researchers found that leg quadriceps muscles were 11 percent stronger in the cyclists who had received massage therapy when compared with the cyclists who had rested for ten minutes.

Whether it is administered before or after exercise, to soothe away muscle soreness, or to help maintain overall muscle health, there's no doubt that massage offers positive benefits for almost every athlete. Let's take a look at how massage helps to maintain overall muscle health.

Muscle Maintenance

When incorporated into an athlete's training schedule, massage is said to promote recovery from intense training, as well as to increase training potential. Regular massage promotes the health of hardworking muscles by improving the circulation of body fluids and by preventing blood from pooling in the capillaries of muscles. Improved circulation also enhances the exchange of substances between blood and tissue cells. In addition, massage helps to decrease swelling in muscle tissues and to stretch and relax sore, overworked muscles—all of which alleviate pain.

Although massage does not directly increase normal muscle strength, it is more effective than rest in promoting recovery from the soreness and fatigue brought on by excessive training or competition. It helps keep your muscles in the best possible state of health and flexibility, so they can function at maximum potential even after recovery from hard exercise.

Pre-Competition Massage

Preparatory massage before competition increases or decreases the excitability of the nerve cells—depending on the type, duration, and intensity of the massage. In addition, supporters of massage say that it warms the muscles, joints, and ligaments, helping to keep them loose and flexible. This protects against injury to cell membranes, often called *microtrauma*.

Pre-competition massage focuses on stretching and warming up the ligaments and tendons of the arms and legs. Because these connective tissues don't have their own blood supply, they don't warm up as quickly as muscle tissue. Massage helps to improve circulation, which results in increased blood flow to relaxed muscle tissues. This, in turn, results in enhanced blood flow to tendons and ligaments. An added benefit is that massage given prior to competition exerts a purely psychological effect by helping anxious and tense athletes to calm down.

It's best to begin pre-competition massage before the warm-up period. Slow stroking can be used to calm the athlete, while a kneading, tapping, or vibrating stroke should stimulate and warm the muscles. The massage should be followed by stretching and a normal, comprehensive warm-up session.

Post-Competition Massage

Most athletes who have experienced post-competition massage will tell you that nothing feels better when the day is done. The therapist works systematically on the athlete's body, progressing from feet, legs, lower back, up to the shoulders, until all the knots and kinks have been worked out. As the muscles relax and loosen, they become more pliable, enhancing the state of relaxation.

Massage therapy following competition helps to eliminate the effects of muscle fatigue. It relieves sore and tense muscles to some extent, while maintaining flexibility and elasticity in the muscles, tendons, and ligaments. Restorative massage after competition is said to speed muscle recovery two to three times faster than just resting, because it promotes blood flow, which works to carry nutrients and oxygen to muscles for repair, and to carry byproducts of metabolism away from muscles.

Hard exercise causes microtrauma to occur in cells, along with some swelling of the muscle tissues. Massage can help to minimize these consequences, or at least to alleviate any pain that accompanies them. Usually, a combination of deep longitudinal strokes to stimulate blood flow; jostling or shaking to relax the muscles; and cross-fiber massage, which involves rubbing across the muscle, is used to relieve pain and stiffness, and to smooth out trigger points that have flared up due to training or racing.

Allow at least thirty minutes after a hard race for a thorough massage in order to feel fully recovered—physically as well as psychologically. The massage should be given in the evening, about one to one and a half hours after your evening meal. This will leave time for the meal to be partially digested so that blood flow—which is greater to the stomach during digestion—can be directed to the muscles.

Injury Repair

Massage can be beneficial in providing a greater range of muscle movement in injured athletes, and it can also help to speed healing at the site of the injury. In addition, it has a positive psychological effect by relaxing and soothing the athlete, thereby reducing the emotional stress that comes with inactivity.

Despite the benefits of massage, however, Andy Pruitt, Certified Athletic Trainer and Director of Sports Medicine at the Boulder Center for Sports Medicine, advises caution in implementing massage therapy if the athlete has sustained muscle damage. "Massage will only traumatize the injured area further under these conditions," says Pruitt. Therefore, massage should not be applied to injured tissue for forty-eight to seventy-two hours after the initial trauma, and certainly not until the swelling and pain have substantially subsided. The three main contraindications to massage (for injured muscles only) are deep muscle trauma, surface abrasions, and tendonitis.

With the increased blood and lymph movement, massage increases nutrition to joints and muscles while hastening the reduction of swelling and the elimination of accumulated inflammatory waste products. The primary ways that lymph moves through the body is through deep breathing, muscular movement, or massage. Massage pressure can help stimulate the lymphatic vessels when exercise is impossible. It is also beneficial in maintaining muscle tone and delaying muscular atrophy, which may result from time off from training.

SAUNAS

Many aching athletes have experienced the soothing and relaxing benefits that a session in a sauna, or steam bath, can provide. The heat and moisture of the sauna induce perspiration, which helps to cleanse the body of impurities through sweating and relieve aches and pains by speeding up circulation and raising body temperature. While the virtues of the sauna as a miracle treatment may be exaggerated, there is scientific and medical evidence that points to its legitimate beneficial effects.

An early study done by Dr. Herb de Vries at the University of Southern California found that the heat of a sauna relaxes muscles. Dr. de Vries measured the electrical activity in the muscles of several subjects who were taking a sauna. He found that the sauna's heat actually brought about a significant decrease in muscle tension. For the competitive athlete, a reduction in muscle tension encourages relaxation, promotes speedy recuperation, and enhances an overall sense of physical and emotional well-being.

The humid heat of the sauna has also been found to help eliminate some of the byproducts of metabolism. During a long, hard exercise session, an athlete may experience a breakdown of tissue protein to be used for fuel, which increases the body's nitrogen level. Nitrogen is a byproduct of protein breakdown that the body cannot use. It is usually removed from the blood by the kidneys and then excreted in the urine. However, a sauna hastens the elimination of nitrogen through the skin as well. Using a sauna allows faster recovery from long and strenuous training sessions because the kidneys do not have to work as hard to eliminate excess nitrogen.

Research has also shown that repeated sessions in the sauna can be as effective as regular mild exercise in conditioning the cardiovascular system. And, in addition to its countless other benefits, the sauna can aid in acclimation to heat stress. The heat of the sauna stresses the body's cooling mechanisms, and this gradually improves the body's capacity to withstand heat. This is important if you are from a cooler region and are preparing for an event that is to take place in a warmer climate. You can increase your body's ability to function in the heat, so that you'll be ready to compete when you arrive.

A popular misconception about saunas is that they are effective tools for weight loss. While you may burn some calories due to the increased demands put on your body by the heat, any significant drop in body weight is only due to water loss. A few glasses of water after a session will put you right back up in weight.

A few words of caution: If you are pregnant, or if you have heart disease or high blood pressure, it's important to consult your physician before you begin taking saunas. This is because the sauna can increase your heart rate. Also, delay your sauna session if you have the symptoms of any illness. The sauna's heat will place added stress on your body, which is already stressed due to the illness. Finally, don't drink alcoholic beverages immediately before or during a session in the sauna. Alcohol has a diuretic effect, which may increase the risk of dehydration.

To derive the greatest possible benefit from a session in the sauna, take note of the following guidelines:

- Allow plenty of time to ensure a leisurely session for maximum benefit. Divide your session into several shorter intervals with a brief rest period between intervals. Also allow time for a longer rest period after you are through.
- Start with moderate heat, and adjust the temperature when you learn at which point your body is most comfortable.
- Sit or lie down on the lowest shelves at the start of each session, where the air is cooler. From there, you can work your way up to the higher shelves for more intense results.
- Allow at least twenty minutes for the last cooling-down period; this should include a shower. If possible, don't towel off immediately, but let the air dry your skin as you cool off. Some people experience lightheadedness and extreme fatigue after a sauna. After resting, however, these sensations should dissipate.
- Replace fluids after your session in order to bring your body back to its normal state of hydration.

Traditional electric heat saunas use the convection system, which heats up the air in order to heat up your body. These systems require between thirty and sixty minutes to preheat so that the moisture in the air is evaporated and the internal temperature is allowed to rise to the proper range of 180°F to 200°F. Recently, there has been an increase in the sales of saunas that use a radiant form of heat, which heats up the body directly, rather than first heating the air. Radiant heat saunas are more efficient and economical, requiring only ten to fifteen minutes to preheat, and a few cents per hour to operate. Radiant heat saunas allow your body to perspire at lower temperatures of about 105°F to 130°F. This type of sauna is more comfortable, so you'll be able to extend the length of your sessions.

STRETCHING

While watching the coverage of the Tour de France one year on television, I noticed that a commentator remarked on the fluid pedaling movements of experienced cyclists such as Jan Ullrich and Bobby Julich. The announcer was amazed by their ability to pedal effortlessly, even while they took time to stretch their shoulders, lower back, and legs while cycling in the breakaway.

After thousands of training miles, professional cyclists have learned techniques to reduce the minor aches and pains that can result from sitting on their bikes in long road races. But stiff, sore muscles are not the bane of cyclists alone. Any athlete who trains long and hard is especially prone to "exercise rigor mortis," a gradual loss of muscle elasticity, accompanied by an increase in joint stiffness. Therefore, athletes have found it necessary to develop simple stretching techniques that allow them to perform at their maximum capacity while reducing tightness and pain in the lower back, shoulders, neck, face, arms, feet, and legs.

As you ride, row, swim, or strength-train on resistance equipment, your muscles become stronger, but tighter—and this tightness can lead to muscle pain. This is a warning sign that you are experiencing a gradual loss of muscle elasticity and a decrease in joint flexibility. Stretching, which requires no special skill and relatively little time, can help prevent stiff and sore muscles and aid in recovery.

Stretching before your workout will help blood to circulate through your muscles, which will warm them up. It will also increase nutrient flow to tissues and provide a period of adjustment to prepare muscles for the hard work to come. Stretching between exercises or when you change pieces of equipment can relieve muscle tension and postpone fatigue. In addition, stretching after your workout should be part of your comprehensive cool-down period to ensure muscle relaxation and to prevent muscle soreness. Stretching in the post-exercise period also helps to circulate nutrients to muscle tissues and to carry waste products away from the muscles. Best of all, stretching exercises done at any time before, during, or after exercise will help you to maintain flexibility, which decreases your risk of muscle injury and increases your physical efficiency and performance.

Stretching Techniques

A long, sustained stretch known as a *static stretch* is a far superior method of stretching your muscles and the surrounding connective tissue when compared with a *ballistic stretch*, which is a rapid and uncontrolled bouncing stretch. Ballistic stretching is generally not recommended for the general population because the high force and short duration of this technique increases the risk of injury.

You should get used to the feeling of an easy static stretch that's low in intensity and that lasts for fifteen to thirty seconds. A static stretch will cause a slight pulling sensation in the muscle, but it should not be painful. If you stretch correctly, and maintain the easy stretch for enough time, the result will be less tension in the muscles you are stretching.

Stretching Exercises

Figures 18.1 through 18.10 show a general ten-minute program that can be done before, after, or even during your workout. These same stretches can also be used during the competition season to aid with stiffness you may experience after a long, hard workout session.

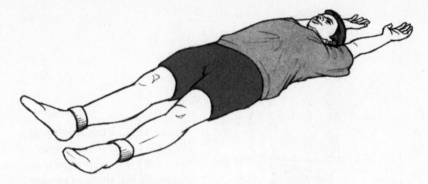

Figure 18.1. Elongation
Straighten out your arms and legs. Point your fingers and toes as you stretch as far as you can. Hold for five seconds, then relax. This is a good way to stretch your entire body.

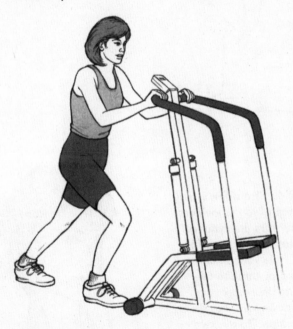

Figure 18.2. Achilles and Calf Stretch
Your back leg should start out straight with the foot flat and pointing straight ahead. Then bend your back knee slightly, still keeping your foot flat. This gives you a much lower stretch, which is good for maintaining or regaining ankle flexibility. Hold for fifteen seconds for each leg. Do not strain the muscles too much—this area needs only a slight sensation of stretching.

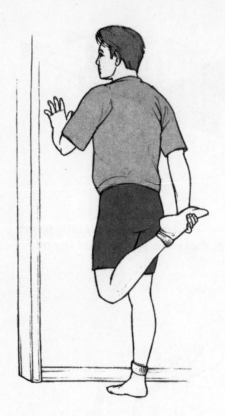

Figure 18.3. Standing Quads
Hold the top of your left foot (on the inside) with your right hand and gently pull the heel toward your buttocks. Repeat with your left hand holding your right foot.

Figure 18.4. Shoulder Shrug
Raise the top of your shoulders toward your ears until you feel slight tension in your neck and shoulders. Hold your shoulders at this point for three to five seconds, and then relax your shoulders downward into their normal position. Do this two or three times. This technique is good to use at the first signs of tightness or tension in the shoulder and neck area.

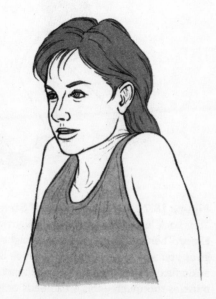

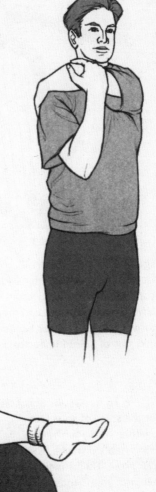

Figure 18.5. Shoulder Stretch
To stretch your shoulder and the middle of your upper back, gently pull your right elbow across your chest toward your opposite shoulder. Hold this position for ten seconds. Repeat with your right elbow.

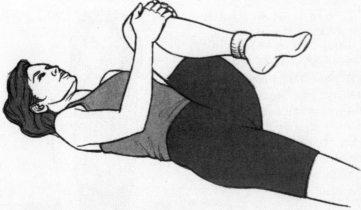

Figure 18.6. Williams Flex Stretch
Straighten both legs and relax, then pull your right leg toward your chest. For this stretch, keep the back of your head on the mat, if possible, but do not strain. Repeat with your left leg.

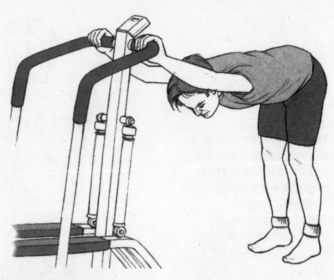

Figure 18.7. Fence Pull
Place both hands shoulder width apart on a ledge and let your upper body drop down as you keep your knees slightly bent. Your hips should be directly above your feet. To change the area of the stretch, bend your knees just a bit more and/or place your hands at different heights. This will take some of the kinks out of a tired upper back.

Figure 18.8. Groin Stretch
Put the soles of your feet together with your heels a comfortable distance from your groin. Then, holding your feet with your hands, slowly pull yourself forward until you feel an easy stretch in the groin. Make your forward movement by bending from the hips, not from the shoulders.

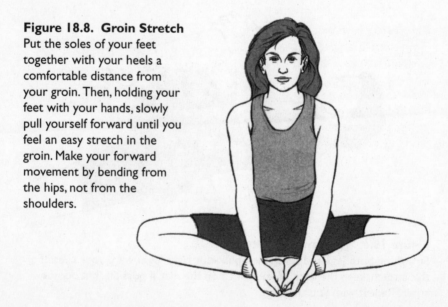

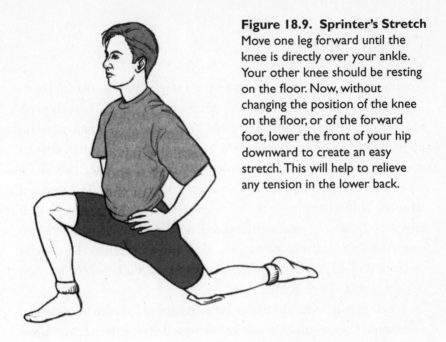

Figure 18.9. Sprinter's Stretch
Move one leg forward until the knee is directly over your ankle. Your other knee should be resting on the floor. Now, without changing the position of the knee on the floor, or of the forward foot, lower the front of your hip downward to create an easy stretch. This will help to relieve any tension in the lower back.

Figure 18.10. Neck Stretch
From a stable, aligned sitting position, turn your chin toward your right shoulder to stretch the left side of your neck. Hold correct stretch tensions for ten to twenty seconds. Stretch each side twice.

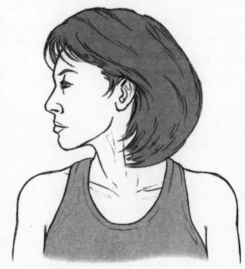

CONCLUSION

Nonnutritional approaches to recovery are as important to overall fitness and muscle recovery as strength and aerobic conditioning. These days, it's not uncommon for athletes to depend on a thorough massage to warm up their muscles before competition or for total body relaxation after an event or training session. Many athletes have also discovered that relaxing in a sauna can work wonders on tired, aching muscles. The heat and moisture of the sauna have been proven to speed up circulation, which increases the flow of vital nutrients to damaged or inflamed muscle tissues. And, in addition to helping the body recover from exercise, these methods double as valuable relaxation time, which is beneficial to emotional health and well-being.

Whether or not you make time for a massage or a session in the sauna, you should always stretch properly before and after exercise. Just a few minutes of simple stretching prior to exercise can help enhance circulation so that your muscles will be warmed up and ready for action. After exercise, stretching ensures proper muscle relaxation and keeps blood flowing at an increased rate to transport nutrients to fatigued and damaged muscle tissues.

The secret to reaching a high level of performance cannot be found in any one food or supplement. Nor does it lie in pushing your body beyond its capacity day after day. *Optimal Muscle Performance and Recovery* has shown you what it has taken many top athletes years to discover: peak performance depends upon paying attention to fuel management during training and competition and optimizing recovery after exercise.

In the last few years, the importance of allowing for recovery time as part of regular training has really come to the forefront. It has been reflected in the design of workout sessions that are less frequent and of shorter duration. Athletes are also being advised to make time for adequate sleep and to take measures to reduce day-to-day stresses. Now, cutting-edge research points to nutrition as an essential piece of the recovery puzzle.

The R[4] System is based on fascinating research that has significantly advanced our understanding of muscle physiology. It incorporates the latest information concerning the need to restore fluids and electrolytes, both during and after exercise. Rehydration is, in fact, the cornerstone of the R^4 System, because sufficient fluid balance is absolutely critical in order to support the body's cardiovascular function and to regulate body temperature. Studies have proven that electrolytes are key factors in facilitating fluid absorption to minimize dehydration.

New information on the importance of the addition of protein to a sports drink during exercise has also been discussed. This new science further enhances muscle performance and reduces the stress of exercise and competition.

Powerful evidence pinpointing insulin's role as the master recovery hormone has been collected from studies conducted at leading universities. These studies have highlighted the importance of consuming key nutrients—most notably, carbohydrate and protein—in the proper proportions within the first two hours after exercise. This stimulates insulin to "kick start" the body's glycogen replenishment and muscle-repair processes.

Scientists and nutritionists have also discovered a connection between strenuous exercise and the buildup of free radicals in the body. Experts now advocate supplementation with antioxidants, including vitamins C and E, in order to minimize free-radical damage, thereby shortening recovery time. Related research into the effects of exercise stress has shown that intense activity compromises the immune system as well, making athletes more susceptible to colds and infections. Natural substances such as glutamine, protein, and even carbohydrate can keep the immune system—and, therefore, the athlete—strong and healthy.

It has been my intention to provide you with some insight into the basic science behind hydration, fuel intake, and muscle support and recovery, in order to give you a head start on improving your individual performance. Although the principles of the R^4 System have grown out of mountains of highly technical scientific evidence, the guidelines for recovery remain simple and practical enough for every athlete to incorporate into training.

Meeting your body's energy needs during and after exercise will give you the strength and endurance you need to reach your long-term goals for training and competition. Your workout doesn't stop when you get off your bike, take off your running shoes, or walk out of the gym. You're not finished until you have refueled and followed the guidelines of the R^4 System to ensure optimal muscle performance and recovery.

Actin. The protein that forms the thin filaments in a muscle fiber.

Adenosine diphosphate (ADP). The molecule formed when one of the phosphate molecules is removed for energy production in the cell.

Adenosine triphosphate (ATP). The source of energy for all living cells.

ADP. See *Adenosine diphosphate.*

Aerobic metabolism. Metabolism in the cell that takes place in the presence of oxygen.

Amino acids. The "building blocks" of proteins. There are 20 different amino acids used by the body.

Anaerobic metabolism. Metabolism in the cell that takes place when there is not sufficient oxygen supplied by the blood to maintain aerobic metabolism.

Antioxidants. Nutrients that seek out and neutralize free radicals in the body, and help the body to recover more quickly from free-radical damage.

ATP. See *Adenosine triphosphate.*

ATP-CP pathway. One of the two anaerobic energy pathways. Energy is released when adenosine triphosphate (ATP) loses one phosphate molecule and becomes adenosine diphosphate (ADP). Creatine phosphate (CP) donates phosphate to replenish ATP stores.

Ballistic stretch. A rapid and uncontrolled bouncing stretch; generally not recommended because of the risk of injury.

Branched-chain amino acids (BCAAs). Amino acids that supply energy by taking the place of glucose in energy pathways; leucine, isoleucine, and valine.

Calories. Units used to measure food energy.

Carbohydrate loading. A nutritional method for delaying fatigue in which the athlete depletes his or her glycogen stores and then consumes a high-carbohydrate diet in the days prior to a competitive event; also known as *glycogen supercompensation.*

Cardiac muscle. The type of muscle that is found only in the heart.

Central fatigue. Fatigue that results from impaired function of the central nervous system; mental fatigue.

Cofactor. A substance that must be present for another substance to be able to perform a particular function.

Complete proteins. Proteins that contain all of the nine essential amino acids.

Complex carbohydrates. Carbohydrates that are composed of long chains of glucose molecules.

Cortisol. A hormone that's released in response to all kinds of stress, including psychological, physical, and emotional stresses.

Creatine phosphate (CP). A molecule in the cell that serves as an energy-producing component.

Creatine kinase (CK). A biochemical marker that is a measure of muscle damage.

Dehydration. The condition caused by excessive loss of water from the body.

Electrolytes. Mineral salts that conduct the electrical energy of the body, and are responsible for muscle contraction and nerve-impulse transmission; sodium, chloride, magnesium, and potassium.

Enzymes. A protein that promotes a chemical reaction without itself being altered in the process.

Ergogenic aid. A nutritional supplement that enhances muscular strength and/or performance.

Essential amino acids. Those amino acids that the body cannot manufacture and that must be supplied by the diet.

Essential fatty acids. Fatty acids that are necessary for rebuilding and producing new cells and maintaining proper brain and nervous-system function.

Fast-twitch muscle fibers. Muscle fibers that contract quickly, providing short bursts of energy; used when strength and speed are needed.

Fatty acids. Components of fat molecules that are used to produce energy.

Foot-strike hemolysis. A condition that occurs because red blood cells are destroyed when the soles of the feet make contact with the hard ground surface.

Free radical. An atom or molecule that is short one electron. It actively seeks out and steals electrons from other parts of the cell.

Glucose. A simple sugar that supplies the body with immediate fuel for energy.

Glutamine. An amino acid that functions as a source of energy for immune cells, and is also readily available for the synthesis of skeletal muscle proteins.

Glycemic index. A measure of the effect of carbohydrate on blood-glucose levels.

Glycogen. A chain of glucose molecules; the form in which glucose is stored in the liver and muscle tissues; it is broken down into glucose for energy when needed.

Glycogen supercompensation. See *Carbohydrate loading.*

Glycogen synthase. An enzyme in the muscle cells that is responsible for converting glucose into glycogen for storage.

Gram (g). A unit of mass. One pound equals 454 grams.

Hemoglobin. The protein responsible for transporting oxygen to muscle cells.

Incomplete proteins. Proteins that are missing one or more of the essential amino acids.

Insulin. A hormone released by the pancreas that helps glucose enter cells from the blood.

International Unit (IU). A unit of weight, usually used for fat-soluble vitamins.

Lactate threshold. The point at which the level of lactic acid in the blood is greater than the body can metabolize.

Lactic acid. A byproduct of anaerobic metabolism that cannot be used effectively by working muscles.

Macronutrients. Nutrients that the body requires daily in large amounts to function properly; water, carbohydrate, fat, and protein.

Microgram (mcg). A unit of mass. A microgram is one-millionth of a gram, or one-thousandth of a milligram.

Micronutrients. Nutrients that are found in the diet and in the body in small amounts; vitamins and minerals.

Microtrauma. Injury to cell membranes.

Milligram (mg). A unit of mass. A milligram is one-thousandth of a gram.

Mitochondria. The structures within cells that are the sites of aerobic energy production.

Myofibrils. The units of muscle fibers that are directly involved in contraction.

Myoglobin. The protein responsible for delivering oxygen from the cell membrane to the mitochondria.

Myosin. The protein that forms the thick filaments in a muscle fiber.

Nonessential amino acids. Amino acids that can be manufactured by the body from other amino acids and therefore do not have to come from the diet.

Osteoporosis. Loss of bone mass or thinning of the bone.

Oxidation. A reaction in which an atom loses an electron.

Rehydration. The process of restoring fluid volumes.

Simple carbohydrates. Carbohydrates that consist of single glucose molecules.

Skeletal muscles. The muscles that cause the movement of bones, also known as *voluntary muscles* and *striated muscles*.

Slow-twitch muscle fibers. Muscle fibers that produce a slow, low-intensity, repetitive contraction and are therefore used for long-term exercise.

Smooth muscle. The type of muscle tissue found in the organs of the digestive system and the walls of blood vessels; also known as *involuntary muscle*.

Sports anemia. A temporary condition resulting from the increase of blood plasma volume, which artificially lowers hemoglobin levels.

Static stretch. A long, sustained stretch that lasts for fifteen to thirty seconds.

Tryptophan. An amino acid that is essential for human metabolism. Tryptophan can cause sleepiness and fatigue when it enters the brain.

CHAPTER 1. HOW MUSCLES WORK

Belanger, A.Y. and A.J. McComas. A comparison of contractile properties in human arm and leg muscles. *European Journal of Applied Physiology* 54 (1985): 26–33.

Campbell, C.J., et al. Muscle fiber composition and performance capacities of women. *Medicine and Science in Sports* 11 (1979): 260–265.

Essen, B.E., et al. Metabolic characteristics of fibre types in human skeletal muscle. *Acta Physiologica Scandinavica* 19 (1975): 153–165.

Gollnick, P.D., et al. Effect of training on enzyme activity and fiber composition of human skeletal muscle. *Journal of Applied Physiology* 34 (1973): 107–111.

Green, J.F. and A.P. Jackman. Peripheral limitations to exercise. *Medicine and Science in Sports and Exercise* 16 (1984): 299–305.

CHAPTER 2. THE ENERGY CURRENCY OF MUSCLES

Chang, T. Wen and A.L. Goldberg. The metabolic fates of amino acids and the formation of glutamine in skeletal muscle. *Journal of Biological Chemistry* 253 (1978): 3685–3695.

Conzolazio, C.F., et al. Protein metabolism during intensive physical training in the young adult. *American Journal of Clinical Nutrition* 28 (1975): 29–35.

DiPrampero, P.E. Energetics of muscular exercise. *Biochemical Pharmacology* 89 (1981): 143–209.

Holloszy, J.O. Adaptation of skeletal muscle to endurance exercise. *Medicine and Science in Sports* 7 (1975): 155–164.

Jacobs, I., et al. Sprint training effects on muscle myoglobin, enzymes, fiber types, and blood lactate. *Medicine and Science in Sports and Exercise* 19 (1987): 369–374.

Karlsson, J. and B. Saltin. Lactate, ATP, and CP in working muscles during exhaustive exercise in man. *Journal of Applied Physiology* 29 (1970): 598–602.

CHAPTER 3. WHAT CAUSES MUSCLE FATIGUE?

Ahlborg, B., et al. Muscle glycogen and muscle electrolytes during prolonged physical exercise. *Acta Physiologica Scandinavica* 70 (1967): 129–142.

Brilla, L.R. and K.B. Gunter. Effects of magnesium supplementation on exercise time to exhaustion. *Medicine, Exercise, Nutrition and Health* 4 (1995): 230–233.

Brouns, F. *Nutritional Needs of the Athlete* (Chichester, Great Britain: John Wiley & Sons, 1993).

Buono, M.J., T.R. Clancy, and J.R. Cook. Blood lactate and ammonium ion accumulation during graded exercise in humans. *The American Physiological Society* (1984): 135–139.

Costill, D.L., et al. Effects of repeated days of intensified training on muscle glycogen and swimming performance. *Medicine and Science in Sports and Exercise* 20 (1987): 249–254.

Costill, D.L., et al. Muscle water and electrolyte distribution during prolonged exercise. *International Journal of Sports Medicine* 2 (1981): 130–134.

Costill, D.L. and M. Hargreaves. Carbohydrate nutrition and fatigue. *Sports Medicine* 13 (1992): 86.

Coyle, E.F. and A.R. Coggan. Effectiveness of carbohydrate feeding in delaying fatigue during prolonged exercise. *Sports Medicine* 5 (1984): 446–458.

Davis, J.M. Carbohydrate, branched chain amino acids and endurance: The central fatigue hypothesis. *Gatorade Sports Science Institute Sports Science Exchange* 9 (1996): 1–6.

Davis J.M. and S.P. Bailey. Possible mechanisms of central nervous system fatigue during exercise. *Medicine and Science in Sports and Exercise* 29 (1996): 45–57.

Konig, D., et al. Zinc, iron, and magnesium status in athletes: Influence on the regulation of exercise-induced stress and immune function. *Exercise and Immunology Review* 4 (1998): 2–21.

Murray, R., et al. The effect of fluid and carbohydrate feedings during intermittent cycling exercise. *Medicine and Science in Sports and Exercise* 19 (1987): 597–604.

Neiman, D.C. Influence of carbohydrate on the immune response to intensive, prolonged exercise. *Exercise Immunology Review* 4 (1998): 64–76.

Newsholme, E.A. Psychoimmunology and cellular nutrition: An alternative hypothesis. *Biological Psychiatry* 27 (1990): 1–3.

Nose, H., et al. Shift in body fluid compartments after dehydration in humans. *Journal of Applied Physiology* 65 (1988): 318–324.

Rudolph, D.L. and E. McAuley. Cortisol and affective responses to exercise. *Journal of Sport Sciences* 16 (1998): 121–128.

Chapter 4. What Causes Muscle Soreness?

Armstrong, R.B. Mechanisms of exercise-induced delayed onset muscular soreness: A brief review. *Medicine and Science in Sports and Exercise* 16 (1984): 529–538.

Armstrong, R.B. Muscle damage and endurance events. *Sports Medicine* 3 (1986): 370–381.

Armstrong, R.B., G.L. Warren, and J.A. Warren. Mechanisms of exercise induced muscle fiber injury. *Sports Medicine* 12 (1991): 184–207.

Evans, W.J. and J.G. Cannon, ed. J.O. Holloszy. *The Metabolic Effects of Exercise-induced Muscle Damage in Exercise and Sport Sciences Reviews* (Baltimore, MD: Williams & Wilkins, 1991), pp. 99–126.

Kanter, M. Free radicals, exercise, and antioxidant supplementation. *International Journal of Sport Nutrition* 4 (1994): 205.

Laursen, P.B. Free radicals and antioxidant vitamins: Optimizing the health of the athlete. *National Strength and Conditioning Association.* 23(2001): 17–25.

Round, J.M., D.A. Jones, and G. Cambridge. Cellular infiltrates in human skeletal muscle: Exercise-induced damage as a model for inflammatory muscle disease. *Journal of Neurological Sciences* 82 (1987): 1–11.

Warholt, M.J., et al. Skeletal muscle injury and repair in marathon runners after competition. *American Journal of Pathology* 118 (1985): 331–339.

CHAPTER 5. RECOVERY: YOUR KEY TO PEAK PERFORMANCE

Hermansen, L., E. Hultman, and B. Saltin. Muscle glycogen during prolonged severe exercise. *Acta Physiologica Scandinavica* 71 (1967):129–139.

Hofman, Z., et al. Glucose and insulin responses after commonly used sport feedings before and after a 1-hour training session. *International Journal of Sport Nutrition* 5 (1995): 194–205.

Thomas, D., et al. Plasma glucose levels after prolonged strenuous exercise correlate inversely with glycemic response to food consumed before exercise. *International Journal of Sport Nutrition* 4 (1994): 361.

CHAPTER 6. REFUEL MUSCLES DURING EXERCISE

Biolo, G., et al. Physiologic hyperinsulinemia stimulates protein synthesis and enhances transport of selected amino acids in human skeletal muscle. *Journal of Clinical Investigation* 95 (1995): 811–819.

Blomstrand E., et al. Administration of branched chain amino acids during sustained exercise: Effects on performance and on plasma concentration of some amino acids. *European Journal of Applied Physiology and Occupational Physiology* 63 (1991): 83–88.

Blomstrand E., et al. Changes in plasma concentrations of aromatic and branch-chain amino acids during sustained exercise in man and their possible role in fatigue. *Acta Physiologica Scandinavica* 133 (1988):115–121.

Blomstrand E., et al. Effect of branched chain amino acid and carbohydrate supplementation on the exercise-induced change in plasma and muscle concentration of amino acids in human subjects. *Acta Physiologica Scandinavica* 153 (1995): 87–96.

Blomstrand E., et al. Effect of branched chain amino acid supplementation on mental performance. *Acta Physiologica Scandinavica* 143 (1991): 225–226.

Blomstrand E., et al. Influence of ingesting a solution of branched chain amino acids on perceived exertion during exercise. *Acta Physiologica Scandinavica* 159 (1997): 41–49.

Blomstrand E., and E.A. Newsholme. Influence of ingesting a solution of branched chain amino acids on plasma and muscle concentrations of amino acids during prolonged submaximal exercise. *Nutrition* 12 (1996): 485–490.

Buchman, A.L., C. Keen, J. Commisso, et al. The effect of a marathon run on plasma and urine mineral and metal concentrations. *Journal of the American College of Nutrition* 17 (1998): 124–127.

Coggan, A.R., and E.E. Coyle. Carbohydrate ingestion during prolonged exercise: Effects on metabolism and performance. *Exercise and Sports Science Review* 19 (1991): 1–40.

Colombani, P.C., et al. Metabolic effects of a protein-supplemented carbohydrate drink in marathon runners. *International Journal of Sport Nutrition* 9 (1999): 181–201.

Davis, J.M., et al. Effects of branched chain amino acids and carbohydrate on fatigue during intermittent, high-intensity running. *International Journal of Sports Medicine* 20 (1999): 309–314.

Esmarck, B., et al. Timing of postexercise protein intake is important for muscle hypertrophy with resistance training in elderly humans. *American Journal of Physiology* 535 (2001): 301–311.

Fahey T.D., et al. The effects of ingesting polylactate or glucose polymer drinks during prolonged exercise. *International Journal of Sport Nutrition* 1 (1991): 249–256.

Flakoll, P.J., et al. Amino acids augment insulin's suppression of whole body proteolysis. *American Journal of Physiology* 257 (1989): E839–E847.

Friden, J., and R.L. Lieber. Structural and mechanical basis of exercise-induced muscle injury. *Medicine and Science in Sports and Exercise* 24 (1992): 521–530.

Galiano, E., et al. Physiologic, endocrine and performance effects of adding branch chain amino acids to a 6 percent carbohydrate-electrolyte beverage during prolonged cycling. *Medicine and Science in Sports and Exercise* 23 (1991): S14.

Halseth, A.E., et al. Effect of physical activity and fasting on gut and liver proteolysis in the dog. *American Journal of Physiology* 273 (1997): E1073–1082.

Hargreaves, M., et al. Effect of carbohydrate feedings on muscle glycogen utilization and exercise performance. *Medicine and Science in Sports and Exercise* 19 (1987): 33–40.

Ivy, J.L., et al. Endurance improved by ingestion of a glucose polymer supplement. *Medicine and Science in Sports and Exercise* 15 (1983): 466–471.

Leatt, P.B. and I. Jacobs. Effect of glucose polymer ingestion on glycogen depletion during a soccer match. *Canadian Journal of Sport Sciences* 14 (1989): 112–117.

Leijssen, D.P.C. Oxidation of exogenous galactose and glucose during exercise. *Journal of Applied Physiology* 79 (1995): 720–725.

Levenhagen, L., et al. Postexercise nutrient intake timing in humans is critical to recovery of leg glucose and protein homeostasis. *American Journal of Physiology* 280 (2001): E982–E993.

Maughan, R.J. Fluid and electrolyte loss and replacement in exercise. *Journal of Sports Sciences* 9 (1991): 117–142.

Mittleman, K.D., et al. Branched chain amino acids prolong exercise during heat stress in men and women. *Medicine and Science in Sports and Exercise* 30 (1998): 83–91.

Murray, R. The effects of consuming carbohydrate-electrolyte beverages on gastric emptying and fluid absorption during and following exercise. *Sports Medicine* 4 (1987): 322–351.

Newsholme E.A., et al. Biochemical mechanism to explain some characteristics of overtraining. In: Brouns, E., ed. *Medical Sports Science Advances in Nutrition and Top Sport* (Basel, Switzerland: Karger), pp. 79–93, 1991.

Nose, H.G., et al. Role of osmolality and plasma volume during rehydration in humans. *Journal of Applied Physiology* 65 (1988): 321–325.

Rehrer, N.J., et al. Effects of electrolytes in carbohydrate beverages on gastric emptying and secretion. *Medicine and Science in Sports and Exercise* 25 (1993): 42–51.

Rennie, M.J., et al. Effect of exercise on protein turnover in man. *Clinical Science* 61(1981): 627–639.

Res, P., et al. The effect of carbohydrate/protein supplementation on endurance performance during exercise of varying intensity. (abstract)

Spiller, G.A., et al. Effect of protein dose on serum glucose and insulin response to sugars. *American Journal of Clinical Nutrition* 46 (1987): 474–80.

Swensen, T., et al. Adding polylactate to a glucose polymer solution does not improve endurance. *International Journal of Sports Medicine.* 15(1994): 430–434.

Tipton, K.D., et al. Postexercise net protein synthesis in human muscle from orally administered amino acids. *American Journal of Physiology* 276 (1999): E628–634.

Tipton, K.D., et al. Timing of amino acid–carbohydrate ingestion alters anabolic response of muscle to resistance exercise. *American Journal of Physiology* 281(2001): E197–E206.

Van Loon, L.J., et al. Plasma insulin responses after ingestion of different amino acid or protein mixtures with carbohydrate. *American Journal of Clinical Nutrition* 72 (2000): 96–105.

Wagenmakers, A.J.M. Role of amino acids and ammonia in mechanisms of fatigue. *Medicine and Sport Science* 34 (1992): 69.

Wasserman, D.H., et al. Interaction of exercise and insulin action in humans. *American Journal of Physiology, Endocrinology and Metabolism* 260 (1991): E37–45.

Yaspelkis, B.B., et al. Carbohydrate supplementation spares muscle glycogen during variable resistance exercise. *Journal of Applied Physiology* 75 (1993): 1477–1485.

Zawadzki, K.M., et al. Carbohydrate/protein supplement increases the rate of muscle glycogen storage post exercise. *Journal of Applied Physiology* 72 (1992): 1854–1859.

CHAPTER 7. REPLENISH GLYCOGEN RAPIDLY

Ahlborg, B., et al. Muscle glycogen and muscle electrolytes during prolonged physical exercise. *Acta Physiologica Scandinavica* 70 (1967): 129–142.

Bergstrom, J., et al. Diet, muscle glycogen and physical performance. *Acta Physiologica Scandinavica* 71 (1967): 140–150.

Biolo, G., et al. An abundant supply of amino acids enhances the metabolic effect of exercise on muscle protein. *American Journal of Physiology* 273 (1997): E122–E129.

Blom, R.C.S., et al. Effect of different post-exercise sugar diets on the rate of muscle glycogen synthesis. *Medicine and Science in Sports and Exercise* 19 (1987): 491–496.

Burke, L.M., G.R. Collier, and M. Hargreaves. Glycemic Index: A tool in sport nutrition. *International Journal of Sport Nutrition* 8 (1998): 401–415.

Burke, L.M., G.R. Collier, and M. Hargreaves. Muscle glycogen storage after prolonged exercise: effect of the glycemic index of carbohydrate feedings. *Journal of Applied Physiology* 75 (1993): 1019–1023.

Copinschi, G., et al. Effect of arginine on serum levels of insulin and growth hormone in obese subjects. *Metabolism* 16 (1967): 485–491.

Costill, D.L., et al. Muscle and liver glycogen resynthesis following oral glucose and fructose feedings in rats. *Biochemistry of Exercise*, Vol. 13, eds. H. Knuttgen, J. Vogel, and J. Poortmans (Champaign, IL: Human Kinetics, 1983), pp. 281–285.

Ivy, J.L., et al. Muscle glycogen storage after different amounts of carbohydrate ingestion. *Journal of Applied Physiology* 65 (1988): 2018–2023.

Ivy, J.L., et al. Muscle glycogen synthesis after exercise: Effect of time of carbohydrate ingestion. *Journal of Applied Physiology* 64 (1988):1480–1485.

Reed, M.J., et al. Muscle glycogen storage postexercise: Effect of mode of carbohydrate administration. *Journal of Applied Physiology* 66 (1989): 720–726.

Roy, B.D., et al. Effect of glucose supplement timing on protein metabolism after resistance training. *Journal of Applied Physiology* 82 (1997): 1882–1888.

Sherman, W.M., et al. Dietary carbohydrate, muscle glycogen, and exercise performance during 7 days of training. *American Journal of Clinical Nutrition* 57 (1993): 27–31.

Spiller, G.A., et al. Effect of protein dose on serum glucose and insulin response to sugars. *American Journal of Clinical Nutrition* 46 (1987): 474–480.

Tarnopolsky, M.A., et al. Postexercise protein-carbohydrate and carbohydrate supplements increase muscle glycogen in men and women. *Journal of Applied Physiology* 83 (1997): 1877–1883.

Varnier, M., et al. Stimulatory effect of glutamine on glycogen accumulation in human skeletal muscle. *American Journal of Physiology* 269 (1995): E309–E315.

Yarasheski, K.E., J.J. Zachwieja, and D.M. Bier. Acute effect of resistance exercise on muscle protein synthesis rate in young and elderly men and women. *American Journal of Physiology* 265 (1993): E210–E214.

Zawadzki, K.M., B.B. Yaspelkis, and J.L. Ivy. Carbohydrate protein complex increases the rate of muscle glycogen storage after exercise. *Journal of Applied Physiology* 72 (1992): 1854–1859.

Chapter 8. Reduce Muscle and Immune-System Stress

Adams, A.K. and T.M. Best. The role of antioxidants in exercise and disease prevention. *The Physician and Sportsmedicine.* 30 (2002): 37–44.

Adibi, S.A. Intravenous use of glutamine in peptide form: Clinical applications of old and new observations. *Metabolism* 38 (supplement 1) (1989): 88–92.

Bassit, R.A., et al. The effect of BCAA supplementation upon the immune response to triathletes. *Medicine and Science in Sports and Exercise.* 32 (2000): 1214–1219.

Bowles, D.K., et al. Effects of acute, submaximal exercise on skeletal muscle vitamin E. *Free Radical Research Communication* 14 (1991):139–143.

Byrnes, W.C., et al. Delayed onset muscle soreness following repeated bouts of downhill running. *Journal of Applied Physiology* 59 (1985): 710–715.

Cannon, J.G., et al. Acute phase response in exercise: Associations between vitamin E, cytokines, and muscle proteolysis. *American Journal of Physiology* 260 (1991): R1235–R1240.

Cannon, J.G., et al. Acute phase response in exercise: Interaction of age and vitamin E on neutrophils and muscle enzyme release. *American Journal of Physiology* 259 (1990): R1214–R1219.

Castell, L.M., et al. The role of glutamine in the immune system and in intestinal function in catabolic states. *Amino Acids* 7 (1994): 231–243.

Castell, L.M., J.R. Poortmans, and E.A. Newsholme. Does glutamine have a role in reducing infection in athletes? *European Journal of Applied Physiology* 73 (1996): 488–490.

Davies, K.J.A., et al. Free radicals and tissue damage produced by exercise. *Biochemical and Biophysical Research Communications* 107(4) (1982): 1198–1205.

Gleeson, M., J.D. Robertson, and R.J. Maughan. Influence of exercise on ascorbic acid status in man. *Clinical Science* 73 (1987): 501–505.

Gohil, K., et al. Vitamin E deficiency and vitamin C supplements: Exercise and mitochondrial oxidation. *Journal of Applied Physiology* 60 (1986): 1986–1991.

Hartmann, A., et al. Vitamin E prevents exercise-induced DNA damage. *Mutation Research* 346 (1995): 195–202.

Hikida, R.S., et al. Muscle fiber necrosis associated with human marathon runners. *Journal of Neurological Sciences* 59 (1983): 185–203.

Hiscock, N. and L.T. Mackinnon. A comparison of plasma glutamine concentrations in athletes of various sports. *Medicine and Science in Sports and Exercise* 30 (1998): 1693–1696.

Jacob, R.A. and B.J. Burri. Oxidative damage and defense. *American Journal of Clinical Nutrition* 63 (1996): 985S–990S.

Keast, D., et al. Depression of plasma glutamine concentration after exercise stress and its possible influence on the immune system. *Medical Journal of Australia* 162 (1995): 15–18.

Lawrence, J.D., et al. Effects of atocopherol acetate on the swimming endurance of trained swimmers. *American Journal of Clinical Nutrition* 28 (1975): 205–208.

Lehmann, M., C. Foster, and J. Keul. Overtraining in endurance athletes: A brief review. *Medicine and Science in Sports and Exercise* 25 (1993): 854–862.

McBride, L.M., et al. Effect of resistance exercise on free radical production. *Medicine and Science in Sports and Exercise* 30 (1998): 67–72.

Meydanit M., et al. Muscle uptake of vitamin E and its association with muscle fiber type. *Journal of Nutritional Biochemistry* 8 (1997): 74–78.

Meydanit, M., et al. Protective effect of vitamin E on exercise induced oxidative damage in young and older adults. *American Journal of Physiology* 264 (1993): R992–R998.

Neiman, D.C. Influence of carbohydrate on the immune response to intensive, prolonged exercise. *Exercise Immunology Review* 4 (1998): 64–76.

Newsholme, E.A. A biochemical mechanism to explain some characteristics of overtraining. *Advances in Nutrition and Topics in Sport* 32 (1991): 79–93.

Newsholme, E.A. Psychoimmunology and cellular nutrition: An alternative hypothesis. *Biological Psychiatry* 27 (1990): 1–3.

Newsholme, E.A. and M. Parry-Billings. Properties of glutamine release from muscle and its importance for the immune system. *Journal of Parenteral and Enteral Nutrition* 14 (1990): 635–675.

Parry-Billings, M., et al. Communicational link between skeletal muscle, brain and cells of the immune system. *International Journal of Sports Medicine* 11 (special supplement) (1990): 1–7.

Quintanilha, A.T. and L. Packer. *Vitamin E, Physical Exercise and Tissue Oxidative Damage in Biology of Vitamin E* (London: E. Pitman, 1983), pp. 56–69.

Robertson, J.D., et al. Increased blood antioxidant systems of runners in response to training load. *Clinical Science* 80 (1991): 611–618.

Rohde, T., K. Krzywkowski, and B.K. Pedersen. Glutamine, exercise, and the immune system: Is there a link? *Exercise Immunology Review* 4 (1998): 49–63.

Rokitai, L., et al. Alpha-tocopherol supplementation in racing cyclists during extreme endurance training. *International Journal of Sport Nutrition* 4 (1994): 253–264.

Rowbottom, D.G., et al. The heternatological, biochemical and immunological profile of athletes suffering from the overtraining syndrome. *European Journal of Applied Physiology* 70 (1995): 502–509.

Rowbottom, D.G., D. Keast, and A.R. Morton. The emerging role of glutamine as an indicator of exercise stress and overtraining. *Sports Medicine* 21 (1996): 80–97.

Sharman, I.M., M.G. Down, and N.G. Norgan. The effects of vitamin E on physiological function and athletic performance of trained swimmers. *Journal of Sports Medicine* 16 (1976): 215–225.

Sharman, I.M., M.G. Down, and N. Sen. The effects of vitamin E and training on physiological function and athletic performance in adolescent swimmers. *British Journal of Nutrition* 26 (1971):265–276.

Shephard, R.J., et al. Vitamin E, exercise and the recovery from physical activity. *European Journal of Applied Physiology* 33 (1974):119–126.

Simon-Schnass, I. and H. Pabst. Influence of vitamin E on physical performance. *International Journal of Vitamin and Nutrition Research* 58 (1988): 49–54.

Stone, M.H., R.E. Keith, J.T. Kearney, et al. Overtraining: A review of the signs, symptoms and possible causes. *Journal of Applied Sport Sciences Research* 5 (1991): 35–50.

Walsh, N.P., et al. Glutamine, exercise and immune function. *Sports Medicine* 26 (1998): 177–191.

CHAPTER 9. REBUILD MUSCLE PROTEIN

Blomstrand, E., et al. Influence of ingesting a solution of branched chain amino acids on plasma and muscle concentrations of amino acids during prolonged submaximal exercise. *Nutrition* (1996):485–490.

Davis, J.M. Carbohydrate, branched chain amino acids and endurance: The central fatigue hypothesis. *Gatorade Sports Science Institute Sports Science Exchange* 9 (1996): 1–6.

Davis, J.M. Carbohydrate, branched chain amino acids, and endurance: The central fatigue hypothesis. *International Journal of Sport Nutrition* 5 (1995): S29–S38.

Davis, J.M. and Bailey S.P. Possible mechanisms of central nervous system fatigue during exercise. *Medicine and Science in Sports and Exercise* 29 (1996): 45–57.

Johnson, D.J., Z.M. Jiang, M. Cotpoys, et al. Branched chain amino acid uptake and muscle free amino acid concentrations predict postoperative muscle nitrogen balance. *Annals of Surgery* 204 (1986): 513–523.

Kreider, R.B., V. Miriel, and E. Bertun. Amino acid supplementation and exercise performance: An analysis of the proposed ergogenic value. *Sports Medicine* 16 (1993): 190–209.

Lemon, P.W.R. Do athletes need more dietary protein and amino acids? *International Journal of Sport Nutrition* 5 (1995): S39–S61.

Madsen, K., et al. Effects of glucose and glucose plus branched chain amino acids or placebo on bike performance over 100 km. *Journal of Applied Physiology* 81 (1996): 2644–2650.

Newsholme, E.A., I.N. Acworth, and E. Blomstrand. Amino acids, brain neurotransmitters and a functional link between muscle and brain that is important in sustained exercise. *Advances in Myochemistry*, ed. G. Benzi (London: John Libbey Eurotext, 1989), pp. 127–133.

Chapter 10. Making Science Practical: The R[4] Recovery System

Boirie, Y. Slow and fast dietary proteins differently modulate postprandial protein accretion. *Proceeding of the National Academy of Sciences USA* 94 (1997): 14930–14935.

Fogt, D.L., J.J. Ivy. Effects of post exercise carbohydrate/protein supplement on skeletal muscle glycogen storage. *Medicine & Science in Sports and Exercise.* 32 (2000): S60.

Ivy, J., et al. Early postexercise muscle glycogen recovery is enhanced with a carbohydrate-protein supplement. *Journal of Applied Physiology* 93 (2002): 1337–1344.

Levenhagen, D.K. et al. Postexercise protein intake enhances whole-body and leg protein accretion in humans. *Medicine and Science in Sport and Exercise* 34 (2002): 828–837.

Ready, S.L., J. Seifert, and E. Burke. Effects of two sport drinks on muscle stress and performance. *Medicine and Science in Sports and Exercise.* 31 (1999): S119.

Roy, B.D., et al. The influence of post-exercise macronutrient intake on energy balance and protein metabolism in active females participating in endurance training. *International Journal of Sport Nutrition and Exercise Metabolism.* 12 (2002): 172–188.

Tipton, K., et al. Exercise, protein metabolism, and muscle growth. *International Journal of Sport Nutrition and Exercise Metabolism.* 12 (2001): 109–132.

Williams, M., J. Ivy, and P. Raven. Effects of recovery drinks after prolonged glycogen-depletion exercise. *Medicine and Science in Sports and Exercise.* 31 (1999): S124.

CHAPTER 11. OPTIMAL RECOVERY FOR THE STRENGTH ATHLETE

Bloomer, J., et al. Effects of meal form and composition on plasma testosterone, cortisol, and insulin following resistance exercise. *International Journal of Sport Nutrition and Exercise Metabolism* 10 (2000): 415–424.

Burke, E. Getting the right amount of protein for endurance and strength training. *Nutrition Science News* 1 (1998): 23–25.

Burke, E.R. MCTs metabolize like carbohydrates. *Nutrition Science News* 12 (1995): 25–27.

Haussinger, E., et al. Cellular hydration state: An important determinant of protein catabolism in health and disease. *Lancet* 341 (1993): 1330–1332.

Houtkooper, L. Nutritional support for muscle weight gain. *NSCA Journal* 8 (1986): 62–63.

Kraemer, W.J., et al. Hormonal responses to consecutive days of heavy-resistance exercise with or without nutritional supplementation. *Journal of Applied Physiology* 85 (1998): 1544–1555.

Kreider, R.B. Dietary supplements and the promotion of muscle growth. *Sports Medicine* 27 (1999): 97–110.

Lemon, P.W.R. Do athletes need more dietary protein and amino acids? *International Journal of Sport Nutrition* 5 (1995): S39–S61.

Levenhagen, D.K., et al. Postexercise protein intake enhances whole-body and leg protein accretion in humans. *Medicine and Science in Sports and Exercise.* 34 (2002): 828–837.

Nissen, S. Effects of HMB supplementation on strength and body composition of trained and untrained males undergoing intense resistance training. Experimental Biology Meeting, Washington, DC, April, 1996.

Pariza, S. Conjugated linoleic acid (CLA) reduces body fat. Experimental Biology Meeting, Washington, DC, April, 1996.

Rasmussen, R., et al. An oral essential amino acid–carbohydrate supplement enhances muscle protein anabolism after resistance exercise. *Journal of Applied Physiology* 88 (2000): 386–392.

Rozenek, R., Stone, M.H. Protein metabolism related to athletes. *NSCA Journal,* 6 (1984): 42–45.

Tipton K.I.D., et al. Postexercise net protein synthesis in human muscle from orally administered amino acids. *American Journal of Physiology* 276 (1999): E628–E634.

Van Loon, et al. Maximizing post exercise muscle glycogen synthesis: carbohydrate supplementation and the application of amino acid or protein hydrolysate mixtures. *American Journal of Clinical Nutrition* 72 (2000): 106–111.

Van Loon, et al. Plasma insulin responses after ingestion of different amino acid protein mixtures with carbohydrates. *American Journal of Clinical Nutrition* 72 (2000): 96–105.

Volek, J.S. and W.J. Kraemer. Creatine supplementation: Its effect on human muscular performance and body composition. *Journal of Strength and Condition Research* 10 (1996): 200–210.

Wolfe, R., et al. Effects of amino acid intake on anabolic processes. *Canadian Journal of Applied Physiology* 26 (2001): 5220–5227.

CHAPTER 12. RECOVERY FOR THE MASTERS ATHLETE

Böhmer, D., et al. Treatment of chondropathia patellae in young athletes with glucosamine sulfate. In: N. Bachl, L. Prokop, and R. Suckert, eds. *Current Topics in Sports Medicine:* 799–900. Vienna, Austria: Urban and Schwarzenberg, 1984.

Bucci, L. *Pain Free: The Definitive Guide to Healing Arthritis, Low-Back Pain, and*

Sports Injuries through Nutrition and Supplements (Fort Worth, TX.: The Summit Group, 1995), pp. 49–77, 117.

Cochran, C. and R. Dent, Cetyl Myristoleate: A Unique Natural Compound Valuable in Arthritis Conditions. *Townsend Letter for Doctors* 168 (1997): 70–74.

Dasa, K., et al. Efficacy of a new class of agents (glucosamine and chondroitin sulfate) in the treatment of an osteoarthritis of the knee. A randomized, double blind, placebo controlled clinical trial. Paper #1 80, 66th annual meeting of the American Academy of Orthopedic Surgeons, Anaheim, California, Feb. 6, 1999.

Jacob, S., R. Lawrence, and M. Zucker. *The Miracle of MSM: The Natural Solution to Pain* (New York, NY, G. P. Putnam's Sons, 1999).

Leffler, C.T., et al. Glucosamine, chondroitin and manganese ascorbate for degenerative joint disease of the knee or low back: A randomized, double-blind, placebo-controlled pilot study. *Military Medicine* 164 (1999): 85–91.

CHAPTER 13. NUTRITION FOR EVERY DAY

Coleman, E. The BioZone nutrition system: A dietary panacea? *International Journal of Sport Nutrition* 6 (1996): 69–71.

Coyle, E.F., et al. Muscle glycogen utilization during prolonged strenuous exercise when fed carbohydrate. *Journal of Applied Physiology* 61 (1986): 165–172.

Coyle, E.F. and S.J. Montain. Benefits of fluid replacement with carbohydrate during exercise. *Medicine and Science in Sports Exercise* 24 (1992): S324–330.

Golay, A., et al. Similar weight loss with low- or high-carbohydrate diets. *American Journal of Clinical Nutrition* 63 (1996): 174–178.

Higher fat 40/30/30 diet fad. *American Running and Fitness Association Running & Fitness News*, 14 (8) (1996): 1.

Karlsson, J. and B. Saltin. Diet, muscle glycogen, and endurance performance. *Journal of Applied Physiology* 31 (1971): 203–206.

Lemon, P.W.R. Effects of exercise on protein requirements. *International Journal of Sport Nutrition* 8 (1998): 426–447.

Lugo M., et al. Metabolic responses when different forms of carbohydrate energy are consumed during cycling. *International Journal of Sport Nutrition* 3 (1993): 398–407.

Sears, B. *The Zone* (New York, NY: HarperCollins, 1995), pp. 40–54.

Sherman W.M., et al. Carbohydrate feedings 1 hr before exercise improves cycling performance. *American Journal of Clinical Nutrition* 54 (1991): 866–870.

Sherman, W. and N. Leenders. Fat loading: The next magic bullet? *International Journal of Sport Nutrition* 5 (1995): S1–S12.

Wright D.A., et al. Carbohydrate feedings before, during, or in combination improves cycling performance. *Journal of Applied Physiology* 71 (1991): 1082–1088.

Young, K., and C.T.M. Davies. Effect of diet on human muscle weakness following prolonged exercise. *European Journal of Applied Physiology* 53 (1984): 81–85.

Young, V.R. and P.L. Pellett. Protein intake and requirements with reference to diet and health. *American Journal of Clinical Nutrition* 45 (1987): 1323–1343.

CHAPTER 14. VITAMINS AND MINERALS: KEYS TO IMPROVED PERFORMANCE

Brilla, L.R. and K.B. Gunter. Effects of magnesium supplementation on exercise time to exhaustion. *Medicine, Exercise, Nutrition and Health* 4 (1995): 230–233.

Cooper, K.H. *Advanced Nutritional Therapies* (Nashville, TN: Thomas Nelson Publishers, 1996).

Cooper, K.H. *Antioxidant Revolution* (Nashville, TN: Thomas Nelson Publishers, 1994).

Gastelu, D. and F. Hatfield. *Dynamic Nutrition for Maximum Performance* (Garden City Park, NY: Avery Publishing Group, 1997).

Karlson, J. *Antioxidants and Exercise* (Champaign, IL: Human Kinetics Publishers, 1997).

Kies, C.V. and J.A. Driskell. *Sports Nutrition: Minerals and Electrolytes* (Boca Raton, FL: CRC Press, 1995).

Konig, D., et al. Zinc, iron, and magnesium status in athletes influence on the regulation of exercise-induced stress and immune function. *Exercise and Immunology Review* 4 (1998): 2–21.

Lieberman, S. *The Real Vitamin and Mineral Book* (Garden City Park, NY: Avery Publishing Group, 1997).

Ulene, A. and V. Ulene. *The Vitamin Strategy* (Berkeley, CA: Ulysses Press, 1994).

Wolinsky, I. *Nutrition in Exercise and Sport* (Boca Raton, FL: CRC Press, 1998).

Wolinsky, I. and J.A. Driskell. *Sports Nutrition* (Boca Raton, FL: CRC Press, 1997).

CHAPTER 15. ENHANCING PERFORMANCE, REDUCING INJURIES, AND IMPROVING RECOVERY WITH SPORTS SUPPLEMENTS

Abraham, W. Factors in delayed muscle soreness. *Medicine and Science in Sports and Exercise.* 9 (1977): 9–20.

Abumrad, N. and P. Flakoll. The efficacy and safety of HMB (Beta-hydroxy-Beta-methylbutyrate) in humans. Vanderbilt University Medical Center, Annual Report: MTI, 1991.

Almada, A., T. Mitchell, and C. Earnest. Impact of chronic supplementation on serum enzyme concentrations. *FASEB Journal* 10 (1996): A4567.

Almada, A., et al. Effects of B-HMB supplementation with and without creatine during training on strength and sprint capacity. *FASEB Journal* 11(3) (1997): A374.

Balsam, R., et al. Creatine supplementation per se does not enhance endurance exercise performance. *Acta Physiologica Scandinavica* 149 (1993): 521–523.

Balsam, P.D., K. Soderlund, and B. Ekblom. Creatine in humans with special reference to creatine supplementation. *Sports Medicine* 18(4) (1994): 268–280.

Böhmer, D., et al. Treatment of chondropathia patellae in young athletes with glucosamine sulfate. In: N. Bachl, L. Prokop, and R. Suckert, eds. *Current Topics in Sports Medicine:* 799–900. Vienna, Austria: Urban and Schwarzenberg, 1984.

Bucci, L. *Pain Free: The Definitive Guide to Healing Arthritis, Low-Back Pain, and Sports Injuries Through Nutrition and Supplements* (Fort Worth, TX.: The Summit Group, 1995), pp. 49–77, 117.

Burke, E. *Creatine: What You Need to Know* (Garden City Park, NY: Avery Publishing Group, 1999).

Burke, E. and T. Fahey. *Phosphatidylserine: Promise for Athletic Performance* (New Canaan, CT: Keats Publishing, 1998).

Burke, L., D. Pyrne, and R. Telford. Effect of oral creatine supplementation on single-effort sprint performance in elite swimmers. *International Journal of Sport Nutrition* 6 (1996): 222–233.

Casal, D.C. and A.S. Leon. Failure of caffeine to affect substrate utilization during prolonged running. *Medicine and Science in Sports and Exercise* 17 (1985): 174–179.

Cheng, W., et al. Beta-hydroxy beta-methylbutyrate increases fatty acid oxidation by muscle cells. *FASEB Journal* 11(3) (1997): A381.

Cichoke, A. *Enzyme & Enzyme Therapy* (New Canaan, CT: Keats Publishing, 1994), pp. 134–148.

Cole, K., D.L. Costill, R. Starling, et al. Effect of caffeine ingestion on perception of effort and subsequent work production. *International Journal of Sport Nutrition* 6 (1996): 14–23.

Costill, D.L., G.P. Dalsky, and W.J. Fink. Effects of caffeine ingestion on metabolism and exercise performance. *Medicine and Science in Sports and Exercise* 10 (1978): 155–158.

DeLanghe, I., et al. Normal reference values for creatine, creatinine, and carnitine are lower in vegetarians. *Clinical Chemistry* 35 (1989): 26–35.

Dietrich, R. Oral proteolytic enzymes in the treatment of athletic injuries: A double blind study. *Pennsylvania Medical Journal* 68 (1965): 35–37.

Dodd, S.L., R.A. Herb, and S.K. Power. Caffeine and exercise performance. *Sports Medicine* 15 (1993): 14–23.

Donaho, C., and C. Rylander. Proteolytic enzymes in athletic injuries. A double-blind study of a new anti-inflammatory agent. *Delaware Medical Journal* 34 (1962): 168–170.

Essig, D., D.L. Costill, and R.J. Van Handel. Effects of caffeine ingestion on utilization of muscle glycogen and lipid during leg ergometer cycling. *International Journal of Sports Medicine* 1 (1980): 86–90.

Fahey, T.D. and M.S. Pearl. The hormonal and perceptive effects of phosphatidylserine administration during two weeks of weight training–induced over-training. *Biological Sport*, in press.

Fisher, S.M., R.G. McMurray, M. Berry, et al. Influence of caffeine on exercise performance in habitual caffeine users. *International Journal of Sports Medicine* 7 (1986): 276–280.

Gaesser, G.A. and R.G. Rich. Influence of caffeine on blood lactate response during incremental exercise. *International Journal of Sports Medicine* 6 (1985): 207–211.

Green, A. Carbohydrate ingestion augments creatine retention during creatine feedings in humans. *Acta Physiologica Scandinavica* 158 (1996): 195–202.

Green, A., et al. Creatine ingestion augments muscle creatine uptake and glycogen synthesis during carbohydrate feeding in man. *Journal of Physiology* 491 (1996): 63.

Hodgdon, J., et al. Plasma hydroxyproline and its association to overuse in training. *Medicine and Science in Sports and Exercise.* 20 (1998): S10.

Hultman, E.K., et al. Muscle creatine loading in man. *Journal of Applied Physiology* 81 (1996): 232–237.

Ivy, J. Effect of pyruvate and dihydroxyacetone on metabolism and aerobic performance. *Medicine and Science in Sports and Exercise* 30 (1998): 837–843.

Ivy, J.L., D.L. Costill, W.J. Fink, et al. Influence of caffeine and carbohydrate feedings on endurance performance. *Medicine and Science in Sports and Exercise* 11 (1979): 6–11.

Kreider, R.B. Creatine supplement: Analysis of ergogenic value, medical safety and concerns. *Journal of Exercise Physiology Online* 1 (1998): 1–11.

Kreider, R., et al. Effects of B-HMB supplementation with and without creatine during training on body composition alterations. *FASEB Journal* 11(3) (1997): A374.

Kidd, P.M. *Phosphatidylserine* (New Canaan, CT: Keats Publishing, 1998).

Monteleone, P., et al. Blunting by chronic phosphatidylserine administration of the stress-induced activation of the hypothalamo-pituitary-adrenal axis in healthy men. *European Journal of Clinical Pharmacology* 41 (1992): 385–388.

Monteleone, P., et al. Effects of phosphatidylserine on the neuroendocrine responses to physical stress in humans. *Neuroendocrinology* 52 (1990): 243–248.

Nissen, S., et al. Effect of leucine metabolite beta-hydroxy-betamethylbutyrate on muscle metabolism during resistance training. *Journal of Applied Physiology* 81 (1996): 2095–2104.

Nissen, S., et al. Effects of feeding beta-hydroxy beta-methylbutyrate (HMB) on body composition in women. *FASEB Journal* 11(3) (1997): A290.

Passwater, R. *Creatine* (New Canaan, CT: Keats Publishing, 1997), pp. 41–42.

Passwater, R. and J. Fuller. *Building Muscle Mass, Performance and Health with HMB* (New Canaan, CT: Keats Publishing, 1997).

Powers, S., R. Byrd, R. Tulley, et al. Effects of caffeine ingestion on metabolism and performance during graded exercise. *European Journal of Applied Physiology* 40 (1983): 301–307.

Spriet, L.L. Caffeine and performance. *International Journal of Sport Nutrition* 5 (1995): S84–S99.

Ternlion, K., et al. The effect of creatine supplementation on two 700-m maximal running bouts. *International Journal of Sport Nutrition* 7 (1997): 138–143.

Thompson, P.D. and B. Franklin. Creatine supplements face scrutiny: Will users pay later? *The Physician and Sportsmedicine* 26 (1998):15–23.

Vanderberghe, K., et al. Caffeine counteracts the ergogenic action of muscle creatine loading. *Journal of Applied Physiology* 80 (1996): 452–457.

CHAPTER 16. NUTRITION TO DELAY EVENT FATIGUE

Anderson, M., et al. Pre-exercise meal affects ride time to fatigue in trained cyclists. *Journal of the American Dietetic Association* 94 (1994): 1152–1153.

DeMarco, H.M., et al. Pre-exercise carbohydrate meals application of glycemic index. *Medicine and Science in Sports and Exercise* 31 (1999): 164–170.

Fairchild, T.J., et al. Rapid carbohydrate loading after a short bout of high intensity exercise. *Medicine and Science in Sports and Exercise* 34 (2002): 980–986.

Piehl, K. Time course for refilling of glycogen stores in human muscle fibres following exercise-induced glycogen depletion. *Acta Physiologica Scandinavica* 90 (1974): 297–302.

Pizza, F., et al. A carbohydrate loading regimen improves high intensity, short duration exercise performance. *International Journal of Sport Science* (1995): 110–116.

CHAPTER 17. SLEEP AND RECOVERY

Brilla, L. R. and V. Conte. A novel zinc and magnesium formulation (ZMA) increases anabolic hormones and strength in athletes. *Sports Medicine and Training Rehabilitation* (In Press), Abstract presented Nov. 14, 1998, at the Annual Meeting of the Southwest Chapter of the American College of Sports Medicine.

Brilla L. R. and V. Conte. Effects of zinc-magnesium formulation increases anabolic hormones and strength in athletes. *Medicine and Science in Sport and Exercise* 31 (1999): S483.

Czeisler, C., et al. Circadian and sleep-dependent regulation of hormone release in humans. *Recent Programs in Hormone Research* 54 (1999): 97–130.

Dement, W. *Can Regular Physical Activity Improve Quality of Sleep in Older Adults?* Stanford, CA: Stanford Center for Research in Disease Prevention, 1994.

Dement, W., and C. Vaughan. *The Promise of Sleep*. New York: Delacorte, 1999.

Di Luigi, L., et al. Acute amino acids supplementation enhances pituitary responsiveness in athletes. *Medicine and Science in Sports and Exercise* 31 (1999): 1748–1754.

Forsling, M., et al. The effect of melatonin administration on pituitary hormone secretion in man. *Clinical Endocrinology.* 51 (1999): 637–642.

Kanaley, J., et al. Cortisol and growth hormone responses to exercise at different times of the day. *Journal of Endocrinology and Metabolism* 86 (2001): 2881–2889.

Kubitz, K.A., D.M. Landers, S.A. Petruzzello, and M. Han. The effects of acute and chronic exercise on sleep: A meta analytic review. *Sports Medicine* 21 (1996): 277–291.

LeDuc, P.A., J.A. Caldwell. A Review of the Relationship among Sleep, Sleep Deprivation, and Exercise. *USAARL Report* 98–25. Fort Rucker, AL. U.S. Army Aeromedical Research Laboratory, 1998.

Mendelson, Wallace. *Human Sleep* (New York: Plenum Press, 1989).

Moore-Ede, M., and S. LeVert. *The Complete Idiot's Guide to Getting a Good Night's Sleep* (New York: Alpha Books, 1998).

Nindl, B., et al. Growth hormone pulsatility profile characteristics following acute heavy resistance exercise. *Journal of Applied Physiology* 91 (2001): 163–172.

Rogers, N., et al. Neuroimmunologic aspects of sleep and sleep loss. *Seminars in Clinical Neuropsychiatry* 6 (2001): 295–307.

Stein T.P., et al. Attenuation of the protein wasting associated with bed rest by branched chain amino acids. *Nutrition* 15 (1999): 656–660.

CHAPTER 18. NONNUTRITIONAL APPROACHES TO RECOVERY

Anderson, B. *Stretching* (Bolinas, CA: Shelter Publications, 1980).

Anderson, B., E. Burke, and B. Pearl. *Getting in Shape: Workout Programs for Men & Women* (Bolinas, CA: Shelter Publications, 1994).

Pozeznik, R. *Massage for Cyclists* (Brattleboro, VT: Vitesse Press, 1995).

INDEX

Achilles and Calf Stretch, 247
Actin, 14
Adipose tissue, 19–21, 26
ADP (adenosine diphosphate), 24, 204
Aerobic metabolism, 23, 34
Aerobic pathway, 25–26
Aging athlete, 149–159
Alanine, 116
Alcohol, and recovery, 56–57
Alpha GPC, 230–231
Amenorrhea, 189
American Journal of Cardiology, 227
Amino acids, 21, 34, 115, 137, 230
    branched-chain, 43, 85–86, 107–108,
        115–117, 177
    essential, 171
    metabolism during exercise, 86
Ammonia, 118–119
Anabolic hormones, 121, 135–136,
        144–145
Anaerobic metabolism, 15, 23

Androgen, 227
Antioxidant Revolution (Cooper), 182
Antioxidants, 101–105, 195, 231
Arginine, 93–94, 127
Arthritis, 155–159
Atherogenic diet, 172
ATP (adenosine triphosphate), 19, 27, 54,
        204–206
ATP-CP pathway, 24

Ballistic stretch, 246
Balsom, Paul, Dr., 204
Bassit, Reinaldo, Dr., 108
B-complex vitamins, 186–187, *186–187*
        table
Biological value (BV), 177
Body temperature, sweating for regulating,
        66
Body-weight composition, 141
Boirie, Y., 129
Boron, 192

Bowerman, Bill, 152
Branched-chain amino acids (BCAAs), 43,
    85–86, 107–108, 115–117, 177,
    230
Brown, Dick, 59
Burke, Louise, Dr., 205

Caffeine, 198–200
Calcium, 42, 188–189
CamelBak hydration system, 74
Capillaries, 14
Carbohydrate, 19–20, 88, 162–163. *See
    also* Carbohydrate loading
  complex, 55
  dietary guidelines for, 163–165
  lowering immune stress with, 110
  for muscle development, 143
  replacement during exercise, 75–79
  sports bars and gels, 165–167
Carbohydrate loading, 1, 6, 29, 215,
    225
  benefits from, 217
  boosting carbohydrate intake, 222–223
  carbohydrate depletion and replenish-
    ment, 216
  classical regimen of, 218
  modified regimen of, 220, *221* table
  new spin on, 221–222
  pre-exercise and pre-event meals,
    223–224
Carbohydrate/protein mixture, 3–4,
    119–120, 136–138, 147–148
Cardiac muscle, 12
Carmichael, Chris, 239
Carotenoids, 184
Cartilage, 155–156, 211
Casein, 129, 178, 230
Catabolic hormones, 135–136
Central fatigue, 43–44
Chloride, 68–69
Cholecystokinin (CCK), 93
Chondroitin, 156
Christensen, E.H., 36
Chromium, 192
Coenzymes, 186
Cofactors, 180
Colds, 111–113
Collagen, 212
Colombani, Paolo, Dr., 79
Contraction, 14
  concentric, 16
  eccentric, 16

Cooper, Kenneth, Dr., 182
Copper, 192–193
Cortisol, 54–55, 110, 115, 136–137, 208,
    229
Costill, David, Dr., 32
Coyle, Edward, Dr., 37, 166
Cramps, muscle, 40–43
Creatine kinase (CK), 104, 127, 139–140,
    207
Creatine monohydrate, 205
Creatine phosphate (CP), 24, 54, 145,
    204–206

Dehydration, 1, 30–31, 41–42
  involuntary, 67
Delayed onset muscle soreness (DOMS),
    39
De Vries, Herb, Dr., 243
Diet: *See also* Nutrition
  atherogenic, 172
  calorie-restricted, 118
  40-30-30, 175–176
  high-carbohydrate, 167
  low-fat, 170
  for master athlete, 153–154
  for strength athletes, 140–144
  typical American, 161
Diuretics, 70
*Dynamic Nutrition for Maximum
    Performance* (Gastelu & Hatfield),
    183

Eccentric contraction, 16
Electrolytes, 191
  adequate ranges in recovery drinks, *132*
    table
  in blood plasma, muscle tissue, and
    sweat, *68* table
  imbalance, 41
  replacement, 67–71, 88
Elongation Stretch, 247
Endurance loss, 113
Endurance sports, 117
Endurance training
  energy production alteration from,
    26–27
  minimizing effects of aging with,
    154
Energy production, 23
  aerobic pathway, 25–26
  alteration of by endurance training,
    26–27

ATP-CP pathway, 24
  glycolysis pathway, 24–25
Energy replacement, 3
Enzymes, 144
Ergogenic aids, 200–203
Estrogen, 189
Evans, William J., Dr., 56, 103
Event fatigue, 215–225
Exercise
  carbohydrate/protein replacement
      during, 21–22, 75–79
  with colds, 111–113
  electrolyte replacement during, 67–71
  fluid replacement during, 73–75
  guidelines for optimum refueling during,
      87–88
  immune system stress from, 101
  protein refueling during for muscle
      protein synthesis, 86–87
  replenishing glycogen after, 91–99

Fahey, Thomas, Dr., 83, 208
Fairchild, Timothy, Dr., 221
Fast protein, 129
Fast-twitch fibers, 14–15, 76
Fat, 20–21, 26, 35, 167
  dietary guidelines for, 169–171
  fatty acids, 168–169
    essential, 169, 179
  for muscle development, 143
Fatigue. *See* Central fatigue; Event fatigue;
      Muscle fatigue; Recovery; Sleep
Fat loading, 219–220
Fat phobia, 167
Fatty acids, 34
Fence Pull Stretch, 250
Ferritin test, 194
Fever, 112
Fiber, 163
Fitness level, 22–23
Fleck, Steven, Dr., 139–140
Fluid
  consumption guidelines, 73–75
  intake, 161–162
  replacement, 66–75, 88–89
4-to-1 ratio carbohydrate/protein drink, 4,
      127–128, 137, 146, 148
Framingham Osteoarthritis Cohort Study,
      157
Free fatty acid, 85
Free radicals, 101
Fructose, 81–82

Galactose, 82
Gastelu, Daniel, 183
Gastric emptying, 73
Gelatin, 157
Gluconeogenesis, 116
Glucosamine, 155–156, 211–212
Glucose, 5, 25, 31, 54, 75
  low blood, 35–37
Glucose-alanine cycle, 116
Glutamine, 106–107, 120–121, 145, 230
Glutathione, 102, 177
Glycemic index, 96–98, 222–223
Glycogen, 5, 19–20, 25, 75, 115
  depletion and fatigue, 34–35
  muscle, 54–55, 84–85
  replenishing after exercise, 91–99, 146
    first hour after, 95
    one to four hours after, 98
    remaining eighteen hours after, 99
  sparing, 23
  storage, 23
  supercompensation, 215
Glycogen synthase, 55, 92
Glycolysis pathway, 24–25
Glycosaminoglycans (GAGs), 212
Goiter, 193
Groin Stretch, 250
Grosman, Mark, Dr., 210
Growth hormone, 136, 228

Hansen, O., 36
Hard-easy training approach, 152
Hatfield, Fred, Dr., 183
HDL (high-density lipoprotein)
      cholesterol, 168
Heavy physical training, 117
Heavy weight training, 118
Heme iron, 194
Hemoglobin, 193
High-carbohydrate diet, 143
HMB, 145, 206–207
Houtkooper, Linda, Dr., 142
Hyponatremia, 71–73

Ibuprofen, 156
IGF-1, 136, 177
Immune system, 56, 229
  and exercise stress, 101
    antioxidants for, 101–105
    supplements for, 106–111
  tips from experts on staying healthy,
      108–109

Inflammation, 212–213
Insulin, 19, 115, 127
  enhancing response of, 93–95
  and glycogen replenishment, 146–147
  role in muscle energy dynamics, 54–55,
    77–78, 88, 92–93
Involuntary dehydration, 67
Iodine, 193
Iron, 193–194
Isoflavones, 178
Isoleucine, 43, 85–86, 108, 115
Ivy, John, Dr., 55, 78–79, 93–94, 117,
    127

Joint pain, 155–159
Journal of Applied Physiology, 128
Julich, Bobby, 245
Junk food, 153

Kearney, Jay T., Dr., 2
Kraemer, William, Dr., 139–140
Kreider, Richard, Dr., 174–175

Lactic acid, 22, 25, 54
  facts and myths about, 38–40
  and muscle fatigue, 37–38
LaLanne, Jack, 151
LDL (low-density lipoprotein) cholesterol,
    168
Leijssen, Dorien, Dr., 82
Leucine, 43, 85–86, 108, 115, 206
Levenhagen, D.K., Dr., 130
Lieberman, Shari, Dr., 182
Liver, 36
Long-term exercise, 2
Lore of Running (Noakes), 58
Low-back pain, 154
Low blood glucose, 35–37

Macronutrients, 18–22, 160. *See also*
    Micronutrients
Magnesium, 42, 70–71, 190
Maltodextrins, 80–81
Manganese, 195
Marketing ingredients, 84
Massage, 239–242
Masters athlete recovery, 149–150
  diet needs, 153–154
  metabolic function, 151
  minimizing aging with endurance
    training and strength training, 154

minimizing injuries with recovery time
    and nutrition, 152–153
  muscle mass and physical capacity, 150
  relieving joint pain and arthritis,
    155–159
Maximum aerobic capacity, 22
Meal-replacement powders, 173–175
Medicine & Science in Sports & Exercise,
    108
Melatonin, 236
Metabolic function, 151
Metabolic waste products, 118–119
Micronutrients, 180. *See also* Macro-
    nutrients; Minerals; Vitamins
Microtrauma, 240–241
Minerals, 180–181, 231. *See also* individual
    minerals; Vitamins
  defined, 187
  major, 188–191
  new standard for sports nutrition,
    181–183
  trace, 191–196
Mitochondria, 27, 167
Mitosis, 229
Mittleman, Kevin, 86
Molybdenum, 195
Monosaccharides, 163
Moore-Ede, Martin, Dr., 231
Morreale, Pietro, 156
MSM, 158–159, 209–211
Muscle cramps, 40–43
Muscle fatigue, 29
  and central fatigue, 43–44
  from dehydration, 30–31
  from lactic acid buildup, 37–40
  from low blood glucose, 35–37
  from muscle fuel depletion, 34–35
  from overheating, 31–33
  protein and BCAAs for reducing, 84–86
Muscle injury, 138–140
  massage for repair, 242
  minimizing with recovery and nutrition,
    152–153
Muscle mass, 150
Muscles, 11
  calorie needs for developing, 142–143
  cardiac, 12
  energy and fluid needs during exercise,
    55–90
  energy for, 18–28
  massage for maintenance, 240

rebuilding protein in, 114–121
skeletal, 17
   fast-twitch and slow-twitch, 14–15
   structure and function, 12–14
   work as antagonistic pairs, 15–16
smooth, 12
untrained, 118–119
Muscle stress, 100
   exercising with colds, 111–113
   and immune system, 105
      supplements for, 106–111
   oxidative stress
      and free radicals, 101
      minimizing with antioxidants,
       101–105
Myofibrils, 14
Myoglobin, 27, 144, 193
Myosin, 14

Naps, 234
National Research Council (NRC), 181
*National Strength & Conditioning
   Association Journal*, 144, 201
Neck Stretch, 251
Newsholme, Eric, Dr., 43, 85, 106–107
Nieman, David, Dr., 110
Nissen, S., 206
Nitrogen, 243
Noakes, Timothy, Dr., 58
NutraJoint, 157
Nutrition, 160–161. *See also* Diet;
   Minerals; Sports nutrition;
   Supplements; Vitamins
   carbohydrate, 162–165
      sports bars and gels, 165–167
   to delay event fatigue, 215–225
   fat, 167–171
   nighttime, 229–231
   protein, 171–179
   water, 161–162

Omega-3 fats, 169
Omega-6 fats, 169
Optimum Daily Intakes (ODIs), 182
Optimum recovery ratio (OR^2), 93, 127
Osmolality, 81
Osteoporosis, 189
Overheating, 31–33
Overtraining syndrome, 58–60, 107
Oxidation, 101
Oxygen, 14, 25

Painkillers, 155
Performance Daily Intakes (PDIs),
   181–183, 196
Phosphatidylserine, 208–209
Phosphocreatine, 145
Phospholipids, 101
Phosphorus, 190–191
Physical capacity, 150
Phytoestrogens, 178
Polylactate, 82–83
Potassium, 69–70
Protein, 21–22, 26, 171
   activities requiring greater amounts,
      117–119
   branched-chain amino acids, 43,
      107–108, 115–117, 177
   complete, 171
   dietary guidelines for, 172–173
   enhancing synthesis of, 119–120
   fast and slow, 128–130
   as fuel source, 115
   incomplete, 171
   for muscle development, 143–144
   nighttime, 229–230
   rebuilding in muscles, 114–121
   replacement during exercise, 75–79
   supplements, 173–179
   synthesis, 86–87
Protein/carbohydrate mixture, 3–4,
   119–120, 136–138, 147–148
Proteolytic enzymes, 212–213
Pruitt, Andy, 242

Raven, Peter, Dr., 126
Recommended Dietary Allowances
   (RDAs), 159, 181
Recovery: *See also* R^4 Recovery System
   and alcohol, 56–57
   intermediate phase of, 54–55
   longer phase of, 55–56
   for masters athlete, 149–159
   nonnutritional approaches to, 238–252
   overtraining dangers, 58–60
   rapid phase of, 54
   sleep for, 226–237
   sports drink for, 124–125, 131–132
   for strength athlete, 135–148
   supplements for, 197–214
Reference Daily Intakes (RDIs), 182
Rehydration, 54, 127
   after exercise, 88–89

Remodeling, 139–140
REM sleep, 227–228
Resistance training, 135
    maximizing, 145–147
Rozenek, Ralph, Dr., 144
R⁴ Recovery System, 2–3, 122, 253–255
    electrolyte ranges per 12 ounces of
        recovery drink, *132* table
    evidence for, 126–128
    fast and slow proteins, 128–130
    recovery sports drink formula, 124–125
    research studies on, 123
    selecting recovery sports drink, 131

SAMe, 158
Sanchez, Daniel, Dr., 210
Saunas, 242–245
Scott, Dave, 122
Seifert, John, Dr., 126
Selenium, 195
Sherman, Michael, Dr., 165, 220
Shoulder Shrug Stretch, 248
Shoulder Stretch, 249
Skeletal muscle, 17
    fast-twitch and slow-twitch, 14–15
    structure and function, 12–14
    work as antagonistic pairs, 15–16
Skinfold measurement, 141
Sleep, 226–227
    aids for, 234–236
    evening before a race, 236–237
    importance of stages 3 and 4, 228–229
    naps, 234
    nighttime nutrition, 229–231
    optimal environment for, 233
    regular schedule for, 231–232
    stages of, 227–228
Slow protein, 129
Slow-twitch fibers, 14–15, 76
Smooth muscle, 12
Sodium, 31, 68–69
Soy protein, 178–179
Spiller, Gene, 78
Sports anemia, 193
Sports bars and gels, 165–167
Sports nutrition
    new standard for, 181–183
    research on, 6–7
Sports-nutrition drinks, 1–2, 77
    multiple uses for, 122–123
    protein-containing, 84–86

for recovery, 124–125
    what to look for in, 80–84
Sprinter's Stretch, 251
Standing Quads Stretch, 248
Static stretch, 246
Stone, Michael, Dr., 144
Strength athlete recovery, 135
    benefits of post-workout supplements,
        136–138
    calorie needs for, 142–143
    carbohydrate and protein before and
        during workouts, 147–148
    carbohydrate/fat needs, 143
    diet for, 140–141
    hormones which alter muscle growth,
        135–136
    maximizing resistance training,
        145–147
    muscle injury, 138–140
    protein needs, 143–144
    supplement needs, 144–145
Stress
    exercise-induced, 101
    minimizing with antioxidants, 101–105
    minimizing with supplements, 106–111
    oxidative from free radicals, 101
Stretching, 245–251
Sulfur, 191
Superoxide dismutase (SOD), 102, 195
Supplements
    for muscle development, 144–145
    post-workout, 136–138
    protein, 173–179
    for recovery, 197–214
    for sleep, 230–231, 234–236
Sweating, 30–31, 66–67
Sweat rate, 74
Swensen, Thomas, Dr., 83

Testosterone, 54, 136, 228–229
Thirst drive, 67
Thyroid gland, 193
Triglycerides, 168–169
Tryptophan, 43, 85
Tufts University Health & Nutrition Letter,
    103–104
Type I muscle fibers. *See* Slow-twitch fibers
Type II muscle fibers. *See* Fast-twitch fibers

Ullrich, Jan, 245
Underwater weighing, 141

Untrained muscles, 118–119
Uric acid, 118–119

Valerian, 235
Valine, 43, 85–86, 108, 115
Van Loon, Luc, 78
Viruses, 111
Vitamin A, 184
Vitamin C, 102–103, 157, 187
Vitamin D, 157, 184
Vitamin E, 103–105, 185
Vitamin K, 185
Vitamins, 180–181, 231. *See also* individual
    vitamins; Minerals
  defined, 183
  fat-soluble, 183–185

new standard for sports nutrition,
    181–183
water-soluble, 185–187

Water, 87–88, 161–162
Weather changes, 42
Whey protein, 129, 176–178, 230
Whole-milk products, 171
Williams Flex Stretch, 249
Wolfe, Robert, Dr., 147–148

Yaspelkis, Ben, 78

Zawadzki, K.M., 78
Zinc, 195–196
ZMA, 230